THE ESSENTIAL GUIDE TO DEMENTIA CAREGIVING

70 VITAL TIPS FOR CAREGIVERS TO KNOW

LINDSAY WHITE, CPTA AND DEMENTIA CAREGIVER

CONTENTS

**Being kind to the old man or old woman
you will you one day become.**

A WORD FROM THE AUTHOR

There is hope! A dementia diagnosis is not the end. There are still many enjoyable times and moments yet to be had for you and your loved one. In fact, some of the best.

At the same time there will be a lot of life change. Dementia comes with countless unexpected syndromes, situations, medical equipment and so many things you need to know.

The goal of this book is to help provide you with the essential tools needed for the dementia caregiving journey in a clear, succinct and helpful way. These are tools I would have liked to have known at the start of our journey.

My hope is that by reading this book you will pick up helpful pieces of information that will help you have more successes and avoid troublesome pitfalls as you navigate this new reality.

You can do this. You are not alone.

There are thousands, if not millions, of dementia caregivers around the world. Being a caregiver for your loved one may turn out to be one of the greatest accomplishments of your life. Love changes you.

Be blessed,

Lindsay White

FOUNDATIONS OF DEMENTIA

1

THE TOP 3 MOST COMMON FORMS OF DEMENTIA

S omething strange is going on. Your loved one isn't acting normal. Is it just expected aging or is there something more?

Other people notice and quietly ask questions. People suspect dementia. You finally realize it is time for a doctor visit to see if this is the case.

When going to the doctor, it is helpful to understand the nuances of the most common forms of dementia so that you can give them good information for them to make an appropriate diagnosis. It is important for doctors to make a correct diagnosis as the different types of dementia require different treatments.

The Top 3 Most Common Forms of Dementia

1) Alzheimer's Dementia – Alzheimer's is the leading form of dementia and perhaps the main one most familiar in the world of dementia diagnoses.

Symptoms fall in line with the standard presentations of dementia:

Memory loss

Mood fluctuation

Vision problems

Misplacing objects

Poor judgment and decision making

Challenges with speaking or writing

2) <u>Lewy Body Dementia (LBD)</u> –This dementia is the disease of a protein in the brain called the "Lewy Bodies." Protein deposits form on the Lewy Bodies and affect the brain's chemical messenger system. This causes issues with mobility, communication, hallucinations, and other maladies.

According to the KU school of Medicine, it often initiatives after the use of general anesthesia from a hospitalization. A notable characteristic of LBD is the high level of delusions. Here are some other characteristics that you may observe.

- Fluctuating cognition – Times when your loved one is mentally clear and times when they are not

- Visual disturbances/delusions that often include colorful people, small animals, and images that may be sexually explicit

- Capgras syndrome is the condition where your loved one sees multiples of everyone, including you, the caregiver, but the person they see in front of them is not the "real" son/daughter/spouse.

- The Lewy lean – A notable strong lean in one direction

- REM sleep disorder, difficulty sleeping, combative sleep expressions, wild dreams, and excessive daytime sleepiness

- Muscle rigidity and stiffness of the arms and legs

Changes in walking and feet movement similar to Parkinson's disease, making them more prone to falls

As surprising as it may sound, Lewy Body Dementia is the second most common form of dementia and growing. One challenge is that it can be so difficult to determine. Estimates show that 70% of people consult with 3 physicians or more before receiving an accurate diagnosis.

A right diagnosis is important as the medicines prescribed will vary for the different dementias. Case in point, the medicine Haldol (haloperidol) that is regularly prescribed for the other forms of dementia is contraindicated/not advisable for Lewy Body Dementia.

3) Vascular Dementia – This type of dementia results from reduced blood flow to the brain, depriving it of essential nutrients. It accounts for 10% of all cases of dementia.

The most common factor of this form of dementia is often the result of a stroke. Strokes hinder the blood flow in the brain and alter the chemical connections and pathways.

Symptoms include:

- Confusion
- Difficulty speaking or concentrating
- Bladder and/or bowel incontinence
- Agitation
- Hallucinations

4) <u>Parkinson's Disease</u> – While Parkinson's is loosely associated with dementia, it is classified as separate from it. Yet many of those with Parkinson's will tend to get a form of dementia.

Furthermore because of the difficulty of diagnosing certain types of dementia, it is not uncommon for a loved one's initial diagnosis to be Parkinson's disease.

<u>Some unique attributes of Parkinson's Disease:</u>

- Mask-like appearance to their face
- A "stuttering" walk with fast, short steps, which is medically called a "festinating gait"
- Cogwheel rigidity (with resisted movement in the forearm)
- Tremors
- Impaired posture and balance
- Hallucinations
- Increased sensitivity to touch or movement that causes pain
- Inability to stop blinking when lightly tapped on the forehead because of neurological changes in the brain

There are several other forms of dementia, but they are not as common as the ones listed above. When your doctor gives you the diagnosis, it is strongly advised to continue your own research and keep learning about your loved one's specific type of dementia.

Come to know what medicines work and do not work for your loved one's condition. See if their symptoms match with the diagnoses. Discuss these with your doctor.

2

KNOW THE 5 GENERAL STAGES
OF DEMENTIA PROGRESSION

It's dementia. Your doctor confirmed it. And with the diagnoses comes a flood of questions. At the root of them is this: What can I expect?

This is not a simple question for a doctor to answer, as no two people are the same. Also, the type of dementia will affect the outcome of your loved one. Alzheimer's differs from Lewy Body Dementia which is also different from Parkinson's Disease.

So what can you expect? There are approximately 5 general stages of dementia progression.

Symptoms can appear at any point and move up and down between stages because of fluctuation in cognition and symptoms. But here is what might unfold or you may observe in your loved one.

Stage 1: Odd Behavior Stage – This is the beginning stage where family members and others notice something is a bit "off" with the person they know. Your loved one may experience a variety of new symptoms:

- Restless leg syndrome
- Laughter at unusual and inappropriate times
- Difficulty sleeping at night
- Increased fears of things that seem unreasonable
- Fluctuating moods
- Paranoia and accusations of family members
- Changes in smell, vision, hearing

Typically, family members sense something is not right but are unsure. The one with dementia may appear perfectly normal and, at other times, show signs of something not quite right. This can confuse family members. Yet it is a normal part of progression.

Stage 2: Disease Discovery Stage - At this stage, the oddities have reached a level of concern, and doctors are typically consulted by family. Your doctor often makes at this point a diagnosis.

Mild symptoms may begin at this stage.

- Constipation
- Sleeping challenges
- Difficulty finding words (expressive aphasia)
- Difficulty in reading or following Tv programs, an inability to focus
- Increased sadness and depression
- Delusions and hallucinations may begin
- Confusion with daily tasks

At this stage it might be time to tactfully start discussing upcoming points of concern such as getting basic legal and financial matters in place. This is critical to do in the early stages when there is a measure of cognition available. If families wait too late, it might require expensive legal interventions later on.

If it hasn't been done already, the window for making decisions about end-of-life issues is almost closed. Is one practically ready? Are things in place? How does one's end-of-life decisions look like? Are they spiritually ready?

Stage 3: Changes – Dementia at this stage becomes obvious and your loved one needs more intentional care. Caregivers also may need additional resources to deal with the increased demands of caregiving. Symptoms may include

- Stumbling and increased risk for falls requiring equipment to assist
- Mumbling, impaired, and sometimes whispering speech
- Increase in delusions and other syndromes
- Increased and intermittent confusion with simple tasks
- Bladder Incontinence
- Loved one needs help with medications
- Increased paranoia and suspicion of crimes committed against them by friends and family
- Only able to follow basic commands
- Urinary Tract Infections (UTI's) may become more common
- Delusions are strong and troubling
- Heavy lean to one side

Stage 4: High-Level Care – At this point, loved ones require a much higher level of care and need help with transfers and feeding. Your loved one needs 24 hours of supervision. Symptoms may include the following.

- Continuous need of assistance with transfers in and out of their chair, bed, going to the bathroom, and with entering/exiting cars
- Bladder and occasional bowel incontinence means taking initiative to reduce and prevent

- Speech is limited to simple sentences and mumbling is increasing
- Delusions and hallucinations present but can be less troublesome
- Intermittent difficulty with swallowing and at times has episodes of choking
- Continued daytime sleepiness
- Increased rigidity and stiffness in the legs and arms

Stage 5 – End Stage – In the last stage, loved ones are fully dependent. It doesn't mean they will pass away soon, but that they physically and mentally need caregivers at all times.

- They become dependent for all daily activities – eating, drinking, brushing teeth, transfers
- Weight loss becomes apparent
- Skin takes on a crepe-like appearance and bruises more easily
- They are strongly affected by temperature fluctuations of both hot and cold
- Difficulty following simple commands
- Mumbling or no language ability
- Need assistance for movement to avoid pressure ulcers
- Choking becomes more increased
- Fluctuations of cognition may become more extreme

Each of these stages is not a hard, fast rule of how things will unfold for your loved one. They are simply general stages you may expect as possibilities.

How long can you expect each of these stages to last? There are so many factors it is impossible to say. Some stages can last years and others merely months.

Even if someone is in the last stage, they can live a short time or even up to several years. No one can say for certain.

It is the same with the question, "How long can my loved one live with dementia?" Some may live only a few months or a year, while others with this disease can live up to 10-15 years. Medicine, genetics, stage of disease, level of care, and more are all factors.

In trying to anticipate the length of life, in practical matters, financial decisions and other decisions are best made with the possibility of a caregiving journey that may last longer than expected. But in matters of the heart, it is better to prepare for the real possibility that a person may pass away sooner rather than later.

The Dying Stage

With dementia, death usually occurs from a loved one aspirating food or liquid into their lungs and then getting pneumonia. At which point they no longer have the ability to cough or expel the liquid in their lungs. Or it can result from the body just shutting down.

The symptoms can include but are not limited to

- When the ability and desire for food and drink stops
- Heart rate increases and wildly fluctuates
- Oxygen levels wildly fluctuate
- The breathing becomes like a rattle and is often irregular
- Hands and feet become cold
- Lack of consciousness and awareness
- Mottled, purple skin on hands and feet
- The bowels completely empty themselves, not just a bowel movement

At this point, nursing is helpful in dealing with pain issues and making sure the process is as comfortable as possible. Morphine and

Tylenol suppositories are often needed. How long it can take varies from person to person. This nursing most likely happens through hospice.

PRACTICAL REALITIES

3
THE ROLLER COASTER CRAZY

Do you remember hearing about one of Aesop's famous fables called "The Boy Who Cried Wolf"? In this story, a shepherd boy fools the townspeople into thinking that a deadly wolf is attacking their flocks. The townspeople race out breathless to protect their flocks only to find that the shepherd boy was playing a joke on them. The shepherd boy does this over and over and thinks it is hilarious.

One day, though, an actual wolf comes and it attacks the flocks. The shepherd boy frantically runs through the village, trying to sound the alarm. By this time, nobody believes him. They have fallen for his trick one too many times. The result is that the sheep are all killed by the wolf.

This is where we get the common colloquial expression, "Never cry wolf." It is about being careful not to raise false alarms to the point no one believes you anymore.

This story becomes a reality with dementia and its fluctuating cognition and moods. There are some days your loved one is doing so well that you think they may live for years to come.

And then just a few weeks later they are so low, struggling with basic functions and slumped over in such a state that you are sure they will pass away within mere weeks. If not days.

Then only a short time later, they are back in a good place again, laughing and talking. It is a wild, ride of the unknown. One that can be hard on the heart and even on relationships.

Challenging as it is, this up-and-down roller coaster ride lasts throughout the entirety of the disease. It can be an emotional drama for the caregivers. You do not know whether to brace yourself for impending death or think that your loved one has many more years to live. How then are caregivers to prepare themselves emotionally?

One thing that can be helpful is not to panic when things are in a bad place. It may just be a slump. A really low slump. Although it could also be something bad, so keeping in good communication with your doctor matters.

At the same time, when it happens so often, you also have to be careful that you do not become calloused. You don't want the disease to "cry wolf" when something may actually be changing. Problems may exist that are real and need to be addressed.

When your loved one is in a low slump, here are some questions to ask:

- Is your loved one getting enough water and liquids?

- Are they developing any pressure wounds or any wounds that might be infected and require medical attention?

- Is it possible they have a Urinary Tract Infection (UTI)? These can make people act and do things they don't normally do.

- Have they had regular bowel movements?

If you have concerns, call your doctor. In these modern times, you can even email them through a health portal email system that most hospitals now implement. It may be necessary to connect with your doctor, as your loved one may legitimately have a medical issue.

It takes experience learning to know when it is a slump and when it is time to call in help. When in doubt, always connect with your medical provider.

Just understand that the roller coaster is part of the journey. It can be difficult. Your loved is not faking their condition. It is just part of the wild world of dementia.

4

SUPPORTING DIGNITY WITH

We all have a desire to be wanted and needed. It is a terrible thought to feel like we are useless. This is also true for your loved one, even as they are journeying through the trials of dementia.

Asking loved ones to support the family in small ways of contribution dignifies them. This may be simple tasks like being asked to help weed the garden, "working" on the car, cooking a meal, or folding laundry. Think about tasks that your loved one can take part with you that are appropriate for their current ability.

1) The tasks should be tasks you do together. Your loved one typically will not be able to process how to complete a task independently, even if they have done them the entirety of their lives. Anything with multiple steps will be difficult for them. They may even ask (read: obsess about asking) that you write it down on a list.

2) Concentration is limited with dementia. The tasks that you give them to assist you with should be short tasks and few in number. The brain of your loved one has a limited ability to concentrate.

3) <u>Their contribution will typically not be done well or even look good but that is Ok</u>.   They are like a small child who wants to help mom in the kitchen but often are more of a hindrance than a help. But the mom still helps them take part anyway because she loves her child. The goal here is not efficiency or doing the task perfectly. It is about giving your loved one a sense of purpose. Just as they did when you were a child "helping" mom or dad out.

4) <u>Your loved one needs a lot of genuine verbal encouragement</u>. Tell them they did a good job with their help and thank them for their contribution. Be genuine and speak to them as an adult, not like a child. Your loved one needs this verbal encouragement and reassurance to feel like a valued part of the family. This will mean more to them than you realize.

As the disease progresses, your tasks will need to change. Perhaps their helping you in the kitchen is simply them sitting there and you asking their advice on how to do things or have them participate by taste-testing. Maybe they go to "work" with you by driving around in your car to do errands.

Whatever you do, help them feel like a valuable contribution to the family. This gives your loved one a sense of purpose and dignity.

5
TIME TRAVELING

It is helpful for your loved one to create familiarity with things that are important to them. One way you can help them is to transport them to a treasured season in their lives.

It is called "time traveling" in that we take them back to "the good old times" of their lives. There are several ways to do this

1) <u>Play Familiar Music</u>

Are you familiar with the musical preferences of your loved one during their youth? Did it involve hymns? Was it Elvis? Was it other "classics" of the time? Put the music on that was familiar to them when they were growing up and in their twenties, a meaningful time for many people.

It can be surprising how the right music can bring things out of your loved one that you have never seen before. You may even want to sing with them along to the music. Make it fun for both you and them.

<u>Dolls and Dogs for Comfort</u>

There comes a time when it is hard for those with dementia to distinguish reality. For women, holding a realistic-looking doll can give them a sense of being a mother again. Like holding a child.

For men, a stuffed dog may bring back a lot of memories. Especially if the stuffed dog looks like a dog they had while growing up.

Even if your loved one knows the stuffed animal is not real, they can connect with their stuffed animal much like a child does. The sensation of holding something soft and fuzzy can be soothing and help them feel playful again.

Let your loved one make their own decisions about when to engage with the doll or stuffed animal. Don't force them to look at it or touch it as it may not be the right moment.

Offer it to them and if they are not interested, try at a later time. Their engagement may vary depending on what is going on in their brain due to fluctuating cognition.

2) Live Animals

Sometimes animals can be a powerful pull of connection for your loved one. If they had a dog growing up, find a service dog or a calm dog from one of your friends to visit occasionally. Even seeing something like a miniature horse can awaken many memories.

Ask yourself what animals were normal in your loved one's life in their growing-up years. Help them make connections with animals in a safe environment.

Your loved one's strongest memories are the long-term memories from their childhood and early adult years. Find ways to bring back those memories and enjoy "living" with them in those times. They are often special days and special connections that bring joy to your loved one.

6

ACTIVE SOCIALIZING

Active socializing for your loved one still needs to continue even in their dementia. It is important that they spend time with their friends and in their social circles, not necessarily yours. Who do they like to be around? What do they like to do?

This can be a curious endeavor based on people's interaction with your loved one's dementia. Some can treat your loved ones like a zoo animal. But don't let this stop you.

Others truly want to be with your loved one no matter what their state. They have been friends or family of your loved one for years. Those social connections still matter to both parties and help provide life-giving interactions for your loved one. Here are some suggestions:

1) Invite *their* friends over for lunch or coffee

Ask yourself which people do you think your loved one still would enjoy being around. It will be up to you as the caregiver to initiate calling them and inviting them over.

You may even need to be the one that carries the conversation. Even when you do your loved one can still enjoy the familiar presence of family and friends.

During the conversation, talk some but also ask what your loved one thinks. Invite them into the discussion. Help your guests feel comfortable by being at ease yourself.

2) Eating out at Restaurants

Going out to eat can still be a possibility even up to the later stages. You may need to feed them and help them with their meal, and that's fine. If that is the case, find a corner of a restaurant and enjoy your meal together.

Sometimes taste is one of the last pleasures to go so help them enjoy different foods. That and being in a different context can be life-giving.

3) Drive-By Visits

At some point, your loved one may not be able to walk. This doesn't mean that they can no longer visit friends and relatives, but how the visit happens may need to be adapted.

Ask their friend if they would be willing if you came to their house to do a "drive-by visit." Bring along with you a stool that their friend can sit on while talking with your loved one through the window.

Visits like this can still bring a lot of encouragement and life. Think of creative ways for social engagement.

4) Attending Community Events

Communities, especially during the summer months, often have special events such as fairs, parades, and other gatherings. Even though your loved one may have struggles, help them be a part of these community events.

The familiar sounds and smells will bring back memories for them. Assist them with eating foods that are special to the events, such as funnel cakes or shaved ice at a fair. Make it enjoyable for them and you.

Ultimately, your loved one still requires significant social connections. They may or may not be able to interact in the same way. But they still hear and have a level of sensory engagement with their environment.

Make sure it is not just your own social connections that your loved is around but also their social networks. Help them be around their friends, former co-workers and those that love them. The connections and presence of familiar people will help bring fullness to your loved one.

7
NEVER ENOUGH WATER

If there is one thing that truly makes a tremendous difference for your loved one it is water. When they have enough water, their whole person functions better, making it easier on you as the caregiver. When they do not have enough water in their system, they are sluggish, slumped and things can be more difficult to manage for the caregiver.

There's only one problem. Generally speaking, those with dementia are not fond of drinking water. Because of this, we may need to be extra intentional in our efforts.

It takes gentleness, encouragement, and intentionality to help loved ones drink appropriate amounts of water and other liquids. Adding flavoring to drinks can help.

Do whatever it takes to help them get a sufficient intake of water. Your doctor can help with you determine the recommended amount.

Here are some ways to increase your loved one's water intake:

1) <u>Watermelon</u> - Watermelon is 95% water and is something your loved one will likely enjoy. It also can bring back special memories of family reunions and other times of their childhood.

Life hack for quick cubing of the watermelon: Using a knife, make deep horizontally and vertically cuts in the halved watermelon about 1/2 inch apart. Then, if you take a large metal stirring spoon (not an everyday spoon) and scoop out the chunks about 1/2" down, the metal spoon will give you the horizontal cuts you need. Shallow scoops make for shorter pieces. Just scoop out at the size you need and you can have a quick bowl of watermelon.

2) <u>Homemade fruit smoothies</u> - Smoothies are great for several reasons. You can add fruit and water and any other fruits you have available. It not only provided good nutrition but the thickness of the smoothies helps to swallow.

Life Hack: Freeze a bunch of bananas with their skin removed. Add them to a smoothie with whatever fruit you have on hand. Keep it at medium thickness.

If your loved one suffers constipation, throw in a handful of dark, leafy greens such as kale or spinach. They likely won't taste the difference and it can help get their bowels moving again.

3) <u>Sipping water all day long</u> - Keep water in a bottle nearby. As a caregiver, help them take a sip whenever you come near.

Life Hack: Use and re-use individual-sized Gatorade bottles as the plastic is thick enough that it can hold together in the dishwasher for several washes. You still will need to wash the bottles regularly so as not to get a buildup of bacteria, especially on the lids.

---

4) Jelly Drops – In recent years, a new product has come out to help those suffering with dementia to increase their levels of hydration. It is called Jelly Drops (www.jellydrops.com).

They are water-based treats with electrolytes to help your loved one get more hydrated. These are great options, especially in the wintertime when things like watermelon are not as readily available.

Do whatever it takes. Sufficient water is essential to the well-being of your loved one. It will also help you as a caregiver when your loved one is in a better state of mind.

8

ALL THINGS FOOD

Food is a big issue for your loved one and has several components in their health journey. It's about helping them eat healthy, avoid trigger foods and minimize choking at all costs.

Helping your loved one get proper nutrition

Caregivers are often tired, and cooking meals and doing dishes can be exhausting. It is tempting to eat out or eat processed meals. Nutrition, though is important for your loved one and has a direct effect on their behavior and cognition.

One thing you can do to ease the stress of the demands of cooking and caregiving is to do make-ahead meals to freeze. Use divided meal plates and when cooking, make extra-large portions that you can then turn into meals for later on. Sometimes Meals-on-Wheels or Mom's Meals can help although they do mean extra costs.

1) Minimizing sugars

Processed sugars can wreak havoc on your loved one's cognition and behavior. It doesn't mean you don't give them desserts or treats.

These still matter for your loved one. But give them in reduced amounts and especially not in the evenings.

Handling Constipation

Constipation can occur often with your loved one, especially in later stages. In later stages, keep a record of bowel movements. This can be as easy as circling the date on a calendar.

If constipation is suspected, one should make a fruit smoothie with greens as a first line of defense. If constipation persists, a doctor may need to be consulted.

Reducing Choking

As the disease progress in your loved one's mind, choking becomes a genuine threat to life. Aspiration can cause pneumonia and to a depleted bodily system, this can mean trouble.

- Learn to cook foods that are soft. Make more meals with pasta, rice, and beans and more easily chewed proteins such as hamburger. Steak may be too risky.

- Cut up meats into small enough chunks that they do not choke

- Perhaps getting a Dechoker device for your home in case of an emergency

2) Minimizing mucus

In the later stages, dairy products can be a factor that increases mucus production in their mouth and causes increased choking. This can include milk, ice cream, cheese products, and other diary-made staples.

If your loved one has trouble choking at night, these may need to be reduced and other alternatives to be introduced. Consult your doctor about possibilities.

Consult a speech therapist - Speech therapy can help people with swallowing by working on training and offering techniques. Sometimes when a person is elderly, they will get to a point where they have squirrel-like tendencies and store food in their cheeks as they eat. It too, is part of the process. This and things like repeated choking may call for medical intervention from your doctor and speech therapists.

As the dementia progresses, it becomes more and more important to monitor your loved one's ability to chew and swallow food safely. They may come to where their mouth forgets how to open, chew, and even swallow.

As a caregiver, adjust accordingly and work with them by providing the appropriate food that they will need. They also may need assistive tools to eat like a weighted spoon.

9
TAKING THE CAR KEYS AWAY

One thing that many caregivers dread is figuring out how to take the keys away from loved ones who have become unsafe. It is necessary, though. Not just for you, but for others on the road.

You do not want to have your loved one involved in a car crash and then someone comes along and sues you for allowing them to drive when you knew they had dementia. Or worse, your loved one has a crash that leads to the loss of life for others and/or themselves. The devastation can be terrible for everyone involved.

Here's the fundamental challenge with those with dementia: Fluctuating Cognition. There are moments where your loved one may appear lucid, as if they can drive with little problem. When that happens, it may seem encouraging to let them keep driving.

The problem is that cognition with dementia fluctuates and changes. A few hours your loved one may be "normal." Ye a few hours later, the confusion sets in.

As a caregiver who is observing your loved one, it is wise not to make your decision of when to take their keys away based on their good days alone. Consider their overall cognition.

If your loved one is experiencing forgetfulness, dizzy spells, confusion, getting lost, having close calls, wandering out of the lane, or difficulty with road signs, it likely is time to intervene.

Additionally, it should be noted that there are countless "missing" elders whose bodies authorities have discovered in rivers and ponds because they drove with dementia. We will talk about this more later but those with dementia are attracted to bodies of water. Especially with cars.

You, as the caregiver, who is with them all the time, will probably see the warning signs to know when to take the keys away. It is better to err on the side of too early rather than too late.

But how? This can be very hurtful to your loved one. It is not easy.

1) It may or may not involve a conversation. Depending on the cognition of your loved one, they may not be able to handle a conversation. Offer them alternatives when they desire to go somewhere.

2) Let them know you would like to drive them whenever they want to go some place. Make your driving them around as a favor to them. Keep it positive.

3) Place the keys in a place where they cannot find them. This can be critical so they do not go driving on their own initiative and cause an accident when you do not even realize they have left.

If you must have the conversation:

You may want to involve a third party like your doctor who tells them they can no longer drive. Ask your doctor to put it in writing so that when the conversation comes up, you can refer your loved one to what they have written. Having a third party such as a doctor speak directly to your loved one can help ease the pressure on you.

4) Let them know you are going to drive for them and they can go wherever they need. Or you will help them obtain transportation. Affirm to them that they are free to go when they need, but that you will help organize their transportation.

It is natural for loved ones to resist. For them, it feels like the taking away their freedom. Because it is exactly that. Speak compassionately, but allow them to feel their feelings.

Do not feel guilty yourself or take it personally if they respond strongly. Dementia significantly impairs their sense of judgment. It may get ugly. But it is better to err on the side of safety rather than to risk a terrible accident. The wrong person could hold you as the caregiver liable.

SYNDROMES, STAGES
AND MORE

10

DEALING WITH DEPRESSION
AND TEARS

How could this have happened? The world was shocked. On August 11, 2014, the news went out on the airwaves. The famous and funny actor Robin Williams who had entertained millions was dead. He had starred in movies like *Good Will Hunting, Good Morning Vietnam,* and *Mrs. Doubtfire,* and now he was gone.

How? Why? What happened? Everyone wanted to know.

It was grief upon grief when it came out that he had committed suicide. This highly successful actor who had brought such joy ended his life abruptly. Why would he do this?

What many people do not know is that when they conducted the autopsy, they discovered that he had one of the worst cases of Lewy Body Dementia that his doctors had ever observed. They were astounded by his ability to complete his final two movies (*Night at the Museum 3* and *Absolutely Nothing*).

Unfortunately, one symptom of dementia that is notable is intense episodes of depression and sadness. Would Robin Williams still be alive if he did not have dementia? Perhaps. We will never know. They thought he had Parkinson's Disease until after the autopsy.

It is an important reminder of just how severe your loved one's sadness and depression can be with any form of dementia. And how seriously we as caregivers need to take it.

While we cannot cure the overall depression that may occur, there are some things that caregivers can do in the moment.

First and foremost, consult your doctor as there may be prescription medicines that can help. And yes, you do need a doctor's consult, as depression medications can interact with other medications they may be taking.

In matters of situational sadness (and not sustained periods of depression), you can help your loved one in the moment.

- If the conversation is going in a way that brings tears from your loved one, you may simply need to change the topic. This helps refocus the brain on something that isn't so sad. Practice redirection.

- Ask them if they would be interested in helping you with a task such as cooking, laundry, or something else easily accessible they can take part in and be successful. Activities can help redirect their brains.

- Change their environment by taking them outside. It is amazing how being outside in more sunlight can change the situational sadness and gloom they may experience.

- Give them a back rub. Some kind of loving touch can help calm their tears. This can soothe them physically as well as provide comfort in their emotional struggle.

- Take them on a car drive. The movement and vibration of the car can help the brain calm down. Any movement can help such as swinging on a porch swing or taking a ride in a golf cart if you have one. Find a way to create movement that can bring stillness to the brain.

It is highly recommended that you refrain from telling them that their sad events are unfounded and not real. Whatever they are experiencing in their minds is very real to them. They cannot help it nor is it logical. Denying their pain amplifies it.

Just reassure them that things are alright and you will take care of it or the problem they speak about. Keep it general. Then gently redirect them to something else. Whatever creative thing you need to do, do so.

Talk to your doctor about the overall sadness and depression. But while at home, help them deal with the situational sadness in what ways work for your loved one. Be creative.

11

FACING THEIR OVERWHELMING FEARS AND ANXIETIES

I magine it is the middle of the night and you see your house is on fire. You jump out of bed and shout to your spouse and children that the house is on fire.

Get out, now!!

The problem is your family does not believe you. They tell you to stop and grumpily roll over and go back to sleep.

If this was a real situation would your panic escalate because they are not believing you? Or would you go back to bed despite the smoke-filled rooms and the crackling sound of flames?

The truth is, we would all lose our minds if the people we loved did not believe us. We would be even more desperate to warn them of impending danger.

This is what it can feel like for your loved one with dementia. When someone dismisses or mocks their fears, those fears like in the fire scenario get amplified 10x as much and your loved one will go into full panic mode.

For them, it is terrifying. They urgently need someone to

A) Believe them and

B) Take action.

How are caregivers to respond?

It actually does not require much. In fact, this is a scenario where less is more. Simple phrases without details often can do the trick.

"I'll go check on that"

"I'll take care of that"

"I took care of it already"

"We have special people protecting us from that"

It is often the only thing they need to hear. Not much more. Why? Because

A) They feel like they are believed

B) Someone is doing something about whatever it is that is scaring them.

There is typically no need to elaborate on details. Just a simple phrase or action. Although sometimes you may need to leave the room and come back so they feel like someone has actually checked on things.

Even if what they are seeing in their mind isn't real, take your loved one's fears as if they were legitimate. Let them know you will be doing something to help resolve the situation.

The peace they often have as a result of your words and action typically diffuses their fears. And with that lessened fear is lessened agitation which can help you as the caregiver.

12

UNDERSTANDING YOUR LOVED ONE'S NEED FOR REASSURANCE

F ear comes in many forms. As the dementia progresses, your loved one's fear of being left alone and abandoned become very real. Some of that fear is based on reality.

Elder abuse, fraud, and neglect are disturbingly high. That and it is very scary being so helpless and dependent.

Because of this, loved ones often attempt to always be overly pleasing to their caregivers. Caregivers often do not see their efforts as they are just trying to cope with the difficult behaviors.

But if a caregiver talks to them about their difficult behavior or something they have done wrong, the loved one is likely to proclaim, "I didn't do it! I didn't do it!" even if they did. Or even if they fear they did. This is the fear of abandonment in a heartbreaking way.

It is futile to get into an argument, especially if your loved one did do something wrong. They will not understand what they did. Or if they do, the fear of abandonment from doing something wrong will terrify them. Their brain cannot handle that level of fear and it shuts down.

The most beneficial thing you can do for them is to reassure them. Let them know "it's Ok" and something such as "we're not sure who did it but it doesn't matter." Speak calmly and lovingly. Let them know they are not being accused or blamed.

Another part of giving them a sense of safety and reassurance is that your loved one frequently needs to hear words of encouragement. Let them know they are doing a good job at the smallest of tasks. Tell them thank-you when they try to help. Help them feel valued and wanted.

Their need for encouragement is leaky by nature. What that means is that they will require frequent encouragement as previous exhortations can be forgotten. Encouragement needs to come often as the memory as encouragement drips out of their emotional reserves and needs refilling. We are all kind of like that.

In summary, be careful of anything that might come across as accusatory or blaming them even if they did do something incorrectly. Offer sincere encouragement at any change you get and when they help you, tell them thank you. This is not just a good practice to help them but it helps us grow as kind people as well. It's just good for everyone.

13
YOUR BODY LANGUAGE MATTERS MORE THAN YOU KNOW

Communication is critical to those with dementia, and it is something that some family and friends may or may not understand. In the early stages of dementia, it is likely that a person can still communicate normally, but as the disease progresses, this can change radically.

One of the biggest factors is verbal processing. Your loved one may or may not understand the full gist of what you are saying. Especially if many words are used.

Simple and slow-paced words are more effective. But if your loved one does not understand you, what they often go by is your tone of voice.

If your tone is stressed and frustrated, they are going to become tearful and fearful that they have done something wrong. They cannot understand why you are upset because they do not process the words the same way as they have normally done in the past.

This is especially challenging as caregivers are often exhausted and frustrated that every little thing requires so much more effort. The tone of a caregiver may have an edge on their words that they did not intend just from fatigue. But the loved one receives it as an attack on themselves.

We tend to all struggle when exhausted. Still, there has to be extra intentionality in speaking with gentle, soothing tones to our loved ones. And when the tone is too sharp, it is good to apologize. Apologies still hit the mark.

Speaking in soothing tones though does not mean treating them like a child. They will pick up on this and it will go downhill quickly. The know that tone of voice well and it is belittling.

In a similar way, loving and kind touch is also valuable for your loved one. Their need for touch as a form of communication experiences a high increase.

More hugs, more arms around the shoulder, or simple back scratches and rubs. As you sit beside them on the couch watching tv, try to connect with them in a way that is comfortable for both of you. Their need for reassuring touch is a good way to communicate non-verbally when done in an appropriate way.

In general, the normal forms of processing through speech fade away with disease progression. Almost like becoming an infant, they need the other forms of communication—slow words, kind tone and loving, appropriate touch. These forms of connection communicate at a much richer level.

14

THE INFAMOUS LEWY LEAN

Depending on the type of dementia of your loved, caregivers may notice a heavy lean to one side. This is particularly the case with Lewy Body Dementia. And it's not just a small lean. Sometimes your loved will be completely lay over to one side.

It is not an issue of physical strength or being difficult. It is a neurological repercussion of dementia. You cannot talk your loved one into correcting the lean or "sitting up straight." Instead, it's good to help them with sitting in a more normal position.

1) Use multiple pillows for bracing when they are on a couch, recliner or even in a wheelchair.

2) Use a neck pillow. When you use a neck pillow, it helps decrease the lean in the body by stopping the head from leaning far to one side. This is perhaps one of the best assists for lean reduction.

3) It is good to reduce the lean as pressure sores can form on various parts of the body such as on the hip bone. You will need to perform occasional checks for such wounds, as pressure ulcers can really be problematic. And very difficult to get healed.

Also the lean can stretch out their neck and cause pain that they cannot articulate. You may also want to massage their neck muscles from time to time. Massage may help reduce some of that neck tension.

15

NAVIGATING DELUSIONS, HALLUCINATIONS AND VISUAL DISTURBANCES

Visual disturbances are another hallmark of dementia. Your loved one may see many things. Typically, what they see are highly colorful people, small children or animals, and can even include sexually lewd things from even the most saintly of people.

This is not your loved one being perverse. It is just a part of what comes from the neurological disturbances in the brain.

Delusions vs. Hallucinations

Delusions and hallucinations are different. Although they can be expounded upon medically to no end, the basic factor is that delusions are seeing distortions of what is real. This is similar to looking at the clouds and instead of seeing clouds, you see what looks like an animal from the shape of the cloud.

Hallucinations are seeing something when there is nothing present. It is not a distortion of reality, but a figment of the mind that interjects something into reality. Hallucinations are also likely to be colorful and vivid.

Visual Disturbances

Visual disturbances can be many-fold. Because the eyes do not work the same, someone may see something that is completely distorted similarly as with delusions.

For example, this may happen when trying to spoon-feed your loved one. Their eyes will suddenly see your hand as a gecko or creature coming to attack them. Or a dog trying to lick them. They will jolt back and recoil.

Just be patient and calm and try to bring your spoon towards their mouth at a different angle. Reassure them in a soothing voice that it is just your spoon.

Delusions, hallucinations, and visual disturbances may be small factors, but not always. At times, they can be extremely severe and cause your loved one to race through the house in fear. Or they may want to run away and escape their present location on foot or in a car.

Trying to convince them that their delusions or hallucinations are not real is futile. You just have to work with them and let them know you are going to take care of it. Reassure them you have things under control, you know of the problem and you will take care of it.

Delusions can also happen at night and this can be especially distressing. For the loved one, it is as if they are in a night terror that they cannot escape. Sometimes, they literally feel trapped in a jail.

For the caregivers, it becomes difficult as sleep becomes limited and it sometimes takes hours to get your loved one in a calmer place and not wanting to run away. Sometimes medication can help.

Know that the severity of the delusions, hallucinations, and visual disturbances come and go. While they may always be present in your loved one to a degree, the intensity of these does not last forever. There are better seasons and worse seasons, though a "season" may last for months at a time.

16

SURVIVING CAPGRAS (IMPOSTER) SYNDROME

For Capgras Syndrome, you will likely need to do as Tom Cruise does in the movie Rainmaker. Head out into an isolated territory, scream as loudly as is in you venting your frustration, then come back and get back to caregiving.

Capgras Syndrome is the syndrome where your loved one sees multiples of you, the caregiver, and everyone else. The real person is always the imposter or the substitute. Your loved one wants to know where the "other" of you is at.

What do you do? (Besides screaming and running away in tears).

1) First, remain calm. Breathe. They cannot help it that you are not the" real you."

Sometimes if you step out for a moment and come back in, even introducing yourself and greeting them enthusiastically, then they will see you as you...maybe. It may take several times.

Often with Capgras Syndrome and dementia in general, there are also multiple homes. They want to go to the "real" home.. It is frustrating and troubling to them when they hear, "We ARE home."

One thing you can tell them is that you are going to take them home. Then redirect them to another task or discussion. They will often forget.

If they don't forget, the best thing to do is go on a drive around the block, and as you pull back into your driveway, happily announce, "Look, we are HOME!!" in a celebratory voice.

If it is at nighttime, you may need to take them to another room. Then let them know they need to eat first or to go to the bathroom. Something that will redirect their minds. At other times, this is the root trigger of their fear.

2) Going outdoors helps. Sunshine makes a notable difference.

This can often be one of the most difficult syndromes for caregivers. It honestly can be exhausting. The first few times it is manageable. But when it comes continuously, it can be a real challenge. Hang in there. Typically, it too comes in waves and seasons.

17
AGGRESSION FROM YOUR LOVED ONE

Some loved ones experience high levels of aggression in the later stages of their journey. With others, there is very little. Aggression can look like

- Shouting
- Hitting/Biting
- Throwing Things
- Cursing, even if they never cussed in their life

Questions to Ask Yourself

1) <u>Is it possible that they could have a UTI</u>? If their aggression comes on over the course of a day and persists for more than a few hours, it may be a urinary tract infection. If that is the case, a doctor visit may be necessary to get some antibiotics.

2) <u>Have they started a newer medication</u>? Sometimes the side effects of medications can cause aggression. If they started a new medication within the last 4-8 weeks, ask your doctor if this is a possibility.

3) <u>Is your loved one getting sufficient nutrition</u>? Lack of proper nutrition can affect their brains. Too much processed food, sugars, and other low-quality foods can be a trigger.

4) <u>Does your loved one think you are a stranger</u>? Sometimes, in their paranoia, they may think their spouse or child is a stranger coming to hurt them. Their aggression may be an act of fear.

Act calmly and keep your distance. It may be necessary to step out of the room for a very short bit. Or switch places with another family member in supervising your loved one.

<u>Are they hungry (or thirsty)</u>? You may try offering a light snack to see if that will help them calm down. Sometimes they can get hungry or thirsty but cannot articular their need for food or water.

<u>What are some things you can do</u>?

- <u>DO NOT TRY TO CONTROL THEM PHYSICALLY</u>. This can turn into a real mess with multiple people hurt.

- <u>Give your loved one some space</u>. Keep in a discreet place where you can check on them but also while keeping some distance.

- <u>Don't argue</u>. Arguing with them and trying to convince them their reality is not what they think it is will make things worse.

- <u>Switch caregivers</u>. If it seems you are a "stranger" and your loved one is acting in fear, have another family member watch them for a bit.

- <u>Use distraction</u>. Put some low music on that they enjoy. Work in the kitchen and hum to show yourself happy.

Redirect them to something pleasant. It doesn't always work, but sometimes it's enough to help.

It is possible that aggression is medically related. If it persists, it is an issue with which to connect with your doctor.

They may need to go in and get checked out to make sure it isn't medicine, an infection or another physical malady triggering their aggression.

18

SILENCING SUNDOWNING

S undowning is a phenomenon that happens typically in the evening when the sun is setting. For your loved one it can feel like the jitters on steroids. Sometimes it's strong and sometimes it isn't.

As the sun goes over the horizon, sundowning can turn your loved one into a nervous mess. It typically only lasts a couple of hours, but those couple of hours can be distressing and exhausting for everyone. What are some things that can help?

1) <u>Satisfy the need for motion</u>. During sundowning, there is an acute need for movement. They may be standing, sitting, nervously walking and more just to satisfy that need for motion.

Put them in the car and drive down some scenic roads. Or even use the wheelchair slowly in the yard or on the sidewalk. Gentle bouncing and movement can help satisfy the need for motion in your loved one.

If it is winter or raining and you can't get out, give them a back massage. They need felt motion.

2) <u>Get outside</u>. The light of the outdoors is helpful to the brain in adjusting the circadian rhythm. First thing in the morning, help your loved one transition to the day with natural, outdoor light. At night when sundowning hits or even a little before, take your loved one outside to eat or do some other activity.

3) <u>Explore some natural over-the-counter supplements</u> -_ Bach's Rescue Remedy Natural supplements may help. It is low cost and can help bring calm. The downside of Bach's is that it is 27% alcohol and seems to have side effects 4-5 hours later. Another option is Energetix Fields of Flower. This one is alcohol-free. It is slower working but has barely noticeable side effects.

4) <u>Provide a calm environment</u>. Stress will agitate sundowning. Stress can come from difficult relationships, clutter in the room, lack of sticking to a schedule, hunger, or even dehydration. Take the initiative as the caregiver to reduce stressful influences.

5) <u>Talk to your doctor</u>. Sometimes things like a low dose of mela-tonin can help. Your doctor can help you navigate sundowning as it is very common in all the different dementia.

Sundowning can be a daily part of the caregiver and loved one's health journey. While there remains much research in to under-standing sundowning, we can take measures to reduce its effects.

19
NAVIGATING INCONTINENCE AND UTI'S

Never underestimate the power of how a Urinary Tract Infection (UTI's) can affect your loved one. It can be surprising.

UTI's are not uncommon in those that have dementia. They can happen for several reasons such as shifting hormones, inadequate cleaning of themselves after using the bathroom, a suppressed immune system, hospitalizations with catheters, or other contributing factors.

When someone with dementia gets a UTI, it can be a small response within which you might notice only a few changes, or they can become violent, aggressive, and demonstrate eye-popping behaviors. If your loved one does become aggressive, it may be worth a trip to the doctor just to see if a UTI may be the cause (or something else).

Another sign of a UTI may be a strong odor in their urine. It will have a very distinct smell and if UTI's happen frequently, you will come to recognize it.

So what can you do?

<u>UTI Prevention</u>

Continue to work towards helping your loved one get enough water intake. Low water is hard on the kidneys, but adequate water can help flush them out. This will help with a level of prevention.

- Hormones are a big contributor, especially among women. Hormone replacement therapy may help if UTI's become too frequent (consult your doctor).

- Make sure your loved one's private area is adequately dry and clean, especially after using the bathroom. But be careful that the drying process is not so harsh that it causes skin irritation to delicate areas.

- If they wear briefs, make sure to change them when they become wet. It's important even with briefs that they stay clean and dry.

- As a side note, having briefs and incontinence pads can help protect your furniture during this phase.

If you suspect a UTI, go to the doctor. They will typically prescribe a round of antibiotics. But don't allow a UTI to go unchecked as it can cause damage.

UTI's are often a part of navigating dementia. Be aware that if their behavior changes, it very well could be a UTI. If they are urinating more frequently and/or that the smell of their urine is much stronger than usual, then a doctor visit should be in order.

20

WHAT IS WITH THE PURSE/WALLET THING?

As a caregiver, it is not uncommon to deal with purse/wallet management. It is a stressor for your loved one. You cannot go anywhere or do anything without getting asked dozens of times, "Where's my purse?" or "Where's my wallet?"

"Right Here," you say, trying to control your patience level after having answered the same question for the thousandth time. What is going on with the purse/wallet obsession?

A purse or wallet is the symbol of freedom, safety, security, and purchase power. It is the representation of something bigger than a mere bag or wallet.

Just know that this is common. They need their "normal" things around them to feel safe and secure. We even need these for ourselves.

Imagine going on a trip and not having your billfold or money. It's unsettling. This is what is happening in the brain of your loved one.

Instead of fighting it, just make sure they have their purse or wallet in their hands. Also,it is good if they have some light money in it to make them feel more comfortable. You can even show them the money inside their purse/wallet and reassure them they are covered.

It brings great peace to your loved one to have their purse or wallet nearby and to have some emergency cash. If that's the price of peace, it's a pretty cheap one.

21

SHOWTIME SYNDROME - THE NEMESIS OF CAREGIVERS

I t is a mystery for caregivers across the world. Your loved one is confused, sees things that are not there, is awake all night, is fixated on asking when they can go home even when they are home, they see multiples of you, they wander, they mumble and more. Yet miraculously it can all change in a moment.

When a friend or relative comes, it is like they are instantly healed. They have very few symptoms. They are clear-minded, sociable, laugh easily and interact like normal. Then as soon as your guests person leave, your loved one lapses right back into their state of confusion and dementia behaviors.

???

This can be maddening to the caregiver. It makes it difficult because other family members don't see what the big deal is you are making about their care.

"There's nothing much wrong with her."

"He's fine."

"Why can't you handle it?"

You wonder if your loved one is faking it. But intrinsically, you know they are not.

Welcome to "Showtime Syndrome."

The social part of the brain is the last part of the brain to be affected. Therefore, socially when someone new enters the scene, the social part of their brain activates to meet them on a "normal" level.

It's not a bad thing but it makes the caregivers look like they don't know what they are talking about. That the caregivers are exaggerating the severity of the symptoms. Nothing could be further from reality.

The truth is you are tired. You need help. But you cannot convince others as they don't see any real problems.

Showtime Syndrome is a challenging reality. The more familiar the person taking care of them, the more the dementia symptoms will show themselves.

It's good to accept that others, including family, will just not understand. Unless they enter the challenges of caregiving, they will only see it from the outside.

Be encouraged that there are thousands of caregivers around the world experiencing the same thing. You are not alone. Nor are you crazy.

Also know this: Your loved one isn't faking it. This is just how the brain works.

What can you do about it? Nothing really. Except have many people over and let them enjoy their socialization. If anything, this is proof that socializing is a high need even in their condition.

22

DAY TIME FLUCTUATIONS

I n a single day, a loved one can experience and exhibit very different expressions of the disease. The two main ones are 1) Fluctuating levels of cognition and 2) Fluctuating levels of awareness and awakeness.

Fluctuating Levels of Cognition

There are moments when your loved one is lucid and talking. And then a few hours later they are anything but that. A few hours later, they are lucid again.

Some wrongly assume that the loved one is faking their various levels of cognition, but this is not the case. Fluctuating cognition is normative for the disease. The reason why this happens in the brain is not widely understood. There is still much research to be done.

When there is diminished levels of cognition, it also is often accompanied by lower levels of speech ability. Loved ones may mumble, slur, or speak rapidly with a "sssss" or "shhhhhh" sound. This is normal.

When someone is having limited cognition, it is helpful that the caregiver responds appropriately. If low cognition is detected, conversation typically needs to be more limited in the amount of words used for conversation. Loved ones will also need a greater level of gentleness in tone from their caregivers.

When your loved one's cognition is elevated, this is a good time to engage your loved one in higher levels of conversation. It is sometimes easy to exclude them in family conversations, but make sure they have a part and have their opinion and contribution in a conversation as well. This can help them feel a sense of belonging.

Include them as they are able, even when cognition is lessened. As a caregiver who is with them often, you will grow in having a sense of when more or lesser interaction is beneficial.

Fluctuating Levels of Awareness

With dementia, a loved one will often have excessive daytime sleepiness. They will not sleep deeply during the night much, but rather sleep slightly off and on throughout the day. This is normal and is a part of the dementia journey.

It is Ok to let them sleep, but it is also good at regular intervals of every several hours to have them seated upright. Or in a chair.

The reason is that you want to avoid pressure sores. Too much time in the same position and the bony protrusions on their body can develop open wounds. These can be dangerous if not properly treated. If your loved one gets an open wound, such as a pressure sore, take them to the doctor.

To help prevent getting a sore, every 2-3 hours their position needs to be changed slightly. This is especially true in later stages where they are less mobile. Changing their position slightly every 2-3 hours is not guaranteed to stop a pressure ulcer, but it can make a difference.

One way to help facilitate this is to have them seated in a recliner. If possible, one that has electrical controls is even better, so positional changes can take place more easily and with more than the two angles of fully upright or fully reclined. The change of angle does not need to be substantial, but enough angle of difference that any potential pressure is shifted off a bony part of the body.

Fluctuations in cognition and awareness are normal in dementia. They typically will happen throughout the day and will last several hours. Adjust accordingly and know this will last throughout your loved one's journey.

23
SPEECH ISSUES AND
IMPORTANT MEMORIES

Dementia results from chemical attacks on the brain making speech much more challenging. It can manifest itself in several ways.

<u>Expressive Aphasia</u>

Expressive aphasia is often seen after strokes, but it can also be a symptom of dementia. This is the condition that when someone is trying to speak, but can't remember the words.

We all have this to some degree as we age, but for those with expressive aphasia, it is at a much more severe level. They have trouble expressing the thoughts they want to communicate. Oftentimes they just give up.

Keep working with them as you patiently try to understand what they are saying.

<u>Mumbling and Whispering</u>

As dementia progresses, so does the mumbling and quiet whispering. Your loved one will often speak quietly, whisper fast, and mumble.

Encourage them to talk loud and big. Sometimes with that, they can get the words out.

The caregiver often struggles to comprehend what is being said. Help them out with possible suggestions of what they might be saying.

If you cannot understand, just smile, affirm them, and let them know you can't understand now but you just might later on.

Yes, there may be a time when your loved one just cannot speak anymore. It is a very sad day as one of the most beautiful things to hear is your loved one's voice.

Speech is one of the most powerful forms of human connection. Appreciate it while you have it.

24

PERSECUTION AND
PARANOIA COMPLEX

Caregivers whose loved ones have dementia often experience the following:

- No matter how much you do, at some point, your loved one states you are not doing enough.

- No matter how much you tell them, they may believe someone is stealing from them or out to harm them.

- No matter what you might say, they may think someone is spying on them.

This. Is. Normal.

It's not a frequent occurrence, but it is part of the journey. And caregivers, if they are not aware of these things, can be hurt by them. But it is not your loved one's typical state of being.

When this is happening, it is the buildup on the frontal part of the brain and the amygdala region at the base of the brain. The front part of the brain handles empathy, impulse control, personality, and judgment.

The amygdala on the other hand helps us to regularize our emotions, fears, and anxieties. With dementia, these parts of the brain are under attack causing paranoia and a sense of persecution. It is literally chemical warfare on the brain.

Nothing that you say with words to reason with them is going to change what they believe. You can only reassure them you believe them and are going to help.

Give them the grace they need. Know that it isn't about you. Nor is it some suppressed anger coming out

And yes, this is easier said than done. When you're exhausted and your loved one says you are not doing enough, it's a blow. Or when they accuse you of something you would never do, it's hard not to react.

But let the truth of the situation be what takes precedence in your thinking. If you need to get away for a bit and allow yourself to be hurt, do so. But don't take it out on your loved one. In their normal thoughts and state, they probably would never even think of these things.

25

HANDLING INAPPROPRIATE LAUGHTER IN SOCIAL SETTINGS

You might have noticed this early on. But somehow your loved one laughs at things that are not funny, or socially out of context. This is often one of the first signs that may present itself when someone is in the beginning stages of dementia.

There is no need to be alarmed. It is a normal part of the disease and thank God for it. How can there ever be too much laughter in the world?

If it's just you and your loved one, laugh with them. Ask them what they saw that was funny so you can join them. Don't laugh at them but with the.

But what if it is a social situation? And you notice other people around you getting uncomfortable? It happens.

Again, there is no need to panic. The best thing you can do is to take control of the conversation, smile at your loved one, and then immediately start talking about something else with the group.

You don't even need to explain to the group. They will follow your lead. The group will redirect, but also so will your loved one.

26

TEMPERATURE FEARS

Those with neurological disturbances demonstrate higher levels of temperature fluctuations. Or any person who is older for that matter.

But those with dementia can really suffer in the summer. If they get overheated, panic can set in. Especially if they get too hot just driving around in a car.

Make sure to keep them reasonably cool. The panic of overheating can be strong. It can lead them to search for bodies of water to cool down and that can be fatal.

Similarly, older individuals commonly experience the effects of getting too cold. As the disease progresses and their age increases, older adults lose the fat layer under the skin. This is visible as their skin takes on a crepe-like appearance. It is very thin and often bruises easily.

Help keep your loved one extra warm during winter. Without that fat layer under their skin, they cannot regulate their body temperature the same way as those around them.

In wintertime, hats, gloves, and coats are a must. And at nighttime, ensure that you adequately cover them with appropriate blankets.

Loved ones tend not to panic as much with the cold, but it is no less real to them. They have very low tolerance for temperature fluctuations and caregivers would do well to help them adjust accordingly by monitoring their external environment.

27
WANDERING MATTERS

Wandering can be a genuine danger to your loved one and something that can be challenging to monitor for the caregiver, especially when it happens at night.   There are many factors that can contribute to your loved one feeling the need to wander.

Potential Instigating Factors

- Are they experiencing **fear** caused by delusions they may be experiencing? This may be especially true if they are wandering at night. If so, have them describe their fears and let them know you are going to take care of it for them.

- Do they **need to use the bathroom** and can't remember where it is at? If so, help them to safely get there.

- Are they **hungry or thirsty** and are wandering the house to search for the kitchen? If so, help them find their way to the kitchen and get what they need.

- Are the repeating **familiar patterns** such as going to work or buying groceries? Go with them and help them accomplish that sense of task.

- Are there **specific tasks** they are feeling compelled to do for a sense of safety and security? If this is the case, help them with the task and let them feel it is accomplished.

- Are they **too hot or too cold**? Loved ones lose the fat layer on their skin and sometimes lose the ability to regulate temperature. If so, adjust accordingly.

- Are they **trying to find their way home** as they just want to "go home"? If so, don't try to argue with them that they are home, but let them know you will take them home later. Or if in the daytime, you may want to drive them around the block and return letting them know they are now home.

Even the most familiar tasks can be forgotten based on how dementia affects the brain. Your loved one may simply have a desire that they need fulfilled but are not sure how to do so.

Wandering isn't harmful in and of itself, but it can lead to harm quickly if not supervised. This is especially true with night wandering.

If your loved one is prone to wandering, here are some helpful steps you may want to take.

Preventive Measures

1) Identification: Make sure your loved one has ID on them. They may, without your knowing, get in the car and start driving. Or they may get lost in a crowd.

Make sure they have your number and contact information in case they get lost and someone can help them. They need identification papers in their pocket and maybe even on a medical bracelet.

2) <u>Find the source of their wandering</u> - Talk with them gently and with soothing tones to determine the nature of why they are wandering. Sometimes small gestures can help bring the comfort they need that a problem is resolved, thus reducing their need to wander.

3) <u>Stay with the Person at All Times</u> - If they are in a wandering phase, the last thing you want to do is run into the store to grab something and return to find out your loved one is no longer in the car. This is true at home as well. Keep them within a watchful distance at all times.

4) <u>Create safe spaces</u> - If you have a fence in your yard, it may be a good time to put a lock on the gate. If they think they can still drive whether or not they have a license, you may need to hide the keys.

5) <u>Install motion sensors and alarms</u> - If your loved one has a serious case of wandering, even if it is just to the bathroom at night, install motion sensors that sound an alarm.

6) <u>Invest in elder trackers</u>. There are elder tracking devices that can help you track your loved one in case they wander too far (Links for these are at the end of the book). You can also sometimes use a more cost-effective means by an Airtag necklace although these do have limitations.

What to do if your loved one is missing

Alert all family members and friends and go on an immediate search. Hopefully, they will just be nearby.

If after a short time you cannot find your loved one, you may need to contact your local authorities. They can search and if your loved one isn't found right away, they may try to ping their cell phone if they have one on their person. If they still can't find your loved one, they can issue a "silver alert" and notify the media.

If the car is missing or they are on foot, after searching for areas that are obvious, **proceed immediately to any nearby body of water**. Individuals with dementia are strangely drawn to large bodies of water such as ponds, lakes, and rivers. These can often do turn life-threatening.

Call your bank and credit card company to see if any transactions have been made. If you are not on the account, they probably won't discuss this with you. But if you are on their financial account, you may be able to find clues.

Find familiar places and routes they may be taking. They may think they need to "go to work" or "visit" a friend. Check what any routes that they would know based on the area where they went missing.

DRESSING, EQUIPMENT AND TRANSFERS

28

EQUIPMENT ACQUISITION

Your equipment needs will change throughout the progression of your love one's illness. You do not need to get everything at once. Get what you need when the need arises. There's a list of reviewed equipment at the end of this book to look into.

Having said that, it can become expensive. If you can purchase the necessary equipment, here are some community resources to check into.

- Medical lending libraries exist in many towns

- The Veterans Office or VFW often has lending libraries even if you are not a veteran

- Check your Medicare B benefits if you have them

- Facebook Marketplace is a good place for equipment, but make sure that it is thoroughly cleaned and tested

- Your Local Area Council on Aging may have resources to connect you locally to those who have equipment

- Your hospital's Physical Therapy and Occupational Therapy department often have connections to help those who need equipment

- Contact your local community health department for connections.

Some equipment you will want to buy new. For example a commode is best to buy new for your loved one. And something like a wheelchair may seem simple but it needs to be fitted to your loved one so as not to create sores. But there is a lot of other equipment that used works fine and can help with the cost.

29
PROGRESSION OF TRANSFER EQUIPMENT

Transfers are simply helping your loved one move from one place to another. You will end up doing thousands if not tens of thousands of transfers as a caregiver, depending on how long your loved one lives.

The progression of equipment is typically as follows:

1) Gait Belt - Needed very early

2) Single Point Cane

3) Quad Cane

4) Four-wheeled walker with sitting bench

5) Front Wheel Walker

6) Standard Walker

7) Wheelchair

8) Stand up Lift

9) Hospital Bed

10) Hoyer Lift

The equipment needs will grow as your loved one's health changes. Insurance and medical plans can help with the cost of these.

Some cities have medical equipment lending libraries. These can be good options. The lending libraries often test the equipment for safety and quality before giving it out.

Each of the pieces of equipment serves a different purpose for a different stage in your loved one's journey. But how do you fit and use these pieces of equipment?

30
GETTING YOUR LOVED ONE DRESSED

In the mid to later stages of dementia, loved ones will often need help getting dressed. This seems easy at the time but sometimes it is not always as it looks.

- Your loved one may have stiffness in the arms and legs.

- They also may be confused with how things work and following instructions

- Their fine motor skills may be significantly diminished

Here are some practical suggestions that will help you as the caregiver as you assist them with getting dressed.

<u>Adding a shirt</u>

1) Start with putting the shirt over their head.

2) Then to get their arms through the holes, reach through the outside of the armhole and put your arm through it to the inside.

Find their respective arm and ask them to "shake hands." This is something they will understand as they are familiar with this practice.

3) When you do shake hands, you can then gently pull their arm through the shirt. Repeat on the other side. Then straighten up the shirt in the back so they look good. And tell them they look good so as to make it a positive experience.

Shirt removal

1) Instead of having them pull their arm out one at a time, the easiest way is to have your loved one lean forward.

2) Then grab their shirt at the back and pull it over their head and arms. If they have a buttoned-up shirt, undo the top few buttons, making the space large enough through which their head goes through.

Buttoning a shirt

Since they are more than likely in sitting, start with lining up the buttons at the top and working your way down. This way it is more likely that the shirt buttons line up with one another.

Women's Bras

Your loved one may have put their bra on in a particular way their whole life. If they are able, you can help facilitate the method they have always used.

But in the mid to later stages of dementia, you may need to assist them with a different method that is easier for you. (And in late stages feel free to ditch the thing).

1) Starting from the front, put both arms through the loopholes.

2) Then move to the back and fasten the latches.

3) Come back to the front tucking "the girls" into their rightful place. Make sure it is comfortable for your loved one and there are no wires sticking out.

Adding brief/disposable underpants when their pants and shoes are on.

When incontinence begins, briefs will often be necessary. To remove disposable underwear, have them sit on the toilet. Then you can simply pull at the waist line of the brief until it tears or use child, blunt end scissors to cut them off.

To put their new briefs back on, you can do so without removing their pants or shoes (once you master this you will be grateful).

1) Find out from the manufacturer of your briefs what is the marker for the front and back of the brief. It usually is a faded gray mark or a design element. The instructions should let you know.

2) Next have them sit down and gather their pants down by their ankles.

3) Take the brief and line it up with the appropriate mark. Then put it over one shoe. Next pull the free loop all the way under and up the pant leg

4) Make sure it is lined up in a normal position with the brief facing to the front and the legs holes in their respective positions. At this point one leg will be in the hole and the other leg's brief you will have in your hand.

5) Next, take the second open leg hole, keep it in position, and thread it down the inside of the pant leg of the other leg.

6) Then before putting it goes over the shoe, turn it a half turn forward.

7) Push the brief over the shoe and back up under the pants.

8) Have them stand and pull the briefs and pants back up and they should be in place. Voila.

This takes a little bit of practice and you may need to follow the instructions several times. But once you get it you will be relieved not to have to remove their pants and shoes every time you need to change their briefs.

Socks

In the early stages, a person may be able to put on their own socks with a sock-donning tool. In the mid to later stages this goes away quickly because of a lack of coordination, comprehension, and more. They just need to be helped.

Dressing Safety

When your loved one is getting dressed, either by themselves or with you, it is very easy for them to lose balance. Make sure to have a gait belt around their waist.

It is best to help them get dressed from their bedside. That way if they lose their balance, they can fall onto their bed.

Changing clothes does not seem like an unsafe activity, but because of their loss of core control based on neurological changes, falls with the changes of clothes are not unprecedented. Do what you can to keep your loved one safe making sure there is something to fall back on.

31

BASIC HOW-TO'S OF AMBULATORY EQUIPMENT

There is a right way and a wrong way to use medical equipment. Some pieces of equipment are best with professional fitting so as not to cause other health problems. Others you can do on your own.

Below are listed basic usage but consult with your physical and occupational therapists for professional assistance.

Gait Belt Usage

At some point, a gait belt becomes a necessity. These are especially necessary when your loved one starts to wobble regularly. They will eventually get to where you will likely need to have them wear a gait belt most of the time. Falls are disastrous.

Sometimes wearing a gait belt can be embarrassing for a loved one. It can help to purchase a gait belt that is darker in color so that they stand out less against your loved one's clothes.

How to Rightly Put on a Gait Belt

There are YouTube videos that can help give you direction on properly putting on a gait belt or you can ask your physical and occupational therapists.

Just as a rule of thumb, you do want at least 12" tail or more extra after the gait belt goes around your loved one so that is certain to be secure in case of any slippage. It shouldn't be right at the buckle. Tuck the tail in to the cinched part of the gait belt so that it isn't flopping around on things.

Here are some basics on putting on a gait belt:

1) The teeth of the gait belt should start at the midline of your loved one with the teeth facing away from the patient on the outside of the belt. The teeth should not be toward the patient or next to their body.

2) When putting the gait belt around your loved one, make sure no lines or tubes for other medical equipment is crossed

3) Wrap the belt around their body, then place the belt under the first bracket, over the toothed part, then back through the other side of the bucket. Tighten snugly but not too tight.

4) Then tuck the tail end of the belt somewhere else in the belt in a way that it does not look like a loop to grab onto

How to Use a Gait Belt

The proper way to use a gait belt is to put your hand under the belt when doing a transfer, as if you are holding water in your hand. The reason is if your loved one starts to fall and you are not looking, your hand will automatically grab the gait belt and it will "catch" in your hand. If your hand is on top, it will slip through your fingers because of the weight of the person.

There are a lot of expensive new-style gait belts that have loops around them. While it is nice to have the handles, the loops tend to be vertical and may not be ideal as they have an increased likelihood of slipping out of your hands with an unexpected fall.

Canes

Canes are great in the early stages. Most people start with a single-point cane and that is good. But a "quad cane" is also highly recommended.

A quad cane has 4 points at the base and helps stabilize walking. They are also great as they don't fall over when not in use but stand up on their own.

In general, to properly fit a cane, have your loved one stand with their arms down at their side. The handle of the cane should match the bony part on the outside of the wrist when their arms are at rest.

It will be approximately a 20-degree angle. This is something that a physical or occupational therapist can help you with and confirm the right fit.

How to use a Cane

The correct way to use a cane is to implement it on the strong side of the body. This is the best way to enhance stability and mobility.

Walkers

There are three types of walkers –

1) Standard Walkers with no wheels.

2) Those with front wheels called Front Wheel Walkers (FWW)

3) Walkers with 4 Wheels called Four Wheeled Walkers (4WW)

So which one do you use? It depends on your loved one's balance. A physical therapist can help you determine which is best.

Generally speaking, a Four Wheeled Walker is best for those with a little bit better balance. It offers them the opportunity to sit and rest as well as get around. Loved ones typically like these in the early stages for the ability to sit and store items.

If your loved one's balance is starting to be affected, a Front Wheel Walker might be next. That way the walker can't run away with them as the back legs of the walker create a measure of drag.

If their balance is really an elevated issue, then a walker with no wheels is ideal, although they can be a little bit more difficult to use for some. Because of this it is common to put tennis balls on the bottom of the legs of the walker to help them glide better. You can even buy tennis balls specifically for a walker.

To fit a walker, you do so the same way as with a cane. Have your loved one stand with their arms down at their side. The handle of the walker should match the bony part on the outside of the wrist approximately at a 20-degree angle. Too low and it makes it difficult for your loved one to push. Too high it can aggravate shoulder issues.

Getting canes, walkers, and wheelchairs appropriately fitted does matter. Always consult your physical therapist and primary care provider. Especially if they are going to be used consistently on a long-term basis as you don't want shoulder injuries, sores, or other problems to develop. But with a good fitting device, the right equipment in the right way can help your loved one move around more safely.

32

SUGGESTIONS FOR BATHROOM AND SHOWER EQUIPMENT

Did you know that one of the most frequent places for falls is the bathroom? This can include getting up in the middle of the night and walking to the bathroom. Or it can be from a fall with the bathroom. Getting the right equipment can help reduce falls and incidents of broken bones.

<u>Bathroom Equipment</u>

Your loved one wants privacy which is understandable, but at the same time they may need extra help. Bathroom safety equipment can help with that.

<u>Stool Riser</u> - Choosing the right one for your loved one

As your loved one may experience variations in their strength, a stool raiser may help keep them safe. It typically has a plastic riser with handles. You can also purchase ones that just have handles by the toilet.

<u>Grab Bars</u> - They need to be strong and secure, not just suction cups

Grab bars are great but they cannot be depended upon to fully support a person's weight. With dementia, it is often the case that they heavily rely on grab bars.

Because of this they need to be secured into the studs of a wal. They must be stable and be able to take a lot of weight.

Shower Bench - Which one is best?

A shower bench is very helpful for you and your loved one. It can help them shower much easier and more thoroughly while also providing a stable place for them to be. But which shower bench is best?

The typical shower bench many use is a lightweight one that is small and goes into the shower, but this may not be best in the long run for those with dementia. Your loved one with dementia oftentimes find it difficult to safely raise their leg over the bathtub edge without losing their balance.

A better option is the shower bench that goes both outside and inside the shower. That way your loved one can start by sitting down on the bench outside of the tub, then safety scooting inside the shower.

Bedside Commode - The Best Equipment for the Time

At some point, your loved one may need a bedside or couch-side commode. There are a couple of factors that will matter.

It is key that the commode is stable if bumped or if your loved one does not have good aim when sitting. You do not want a commode that can tip over, especially as those with dementia may have a hard lean to one side. Their needs for stability in a commode are more significant than just the average elderly person.

A bench-style drop-arm commode is a great option. It is more stable, the loved one does not need to be lifted as high and they can scoot over onto the commode. If their aim in sitting is off there is more safety and stability with the bench. A good commode also has a removable bowl area and it can double as a shower bench with its adjustable legs.

Finding the right equipment to increase the safety of your loved one is vital. Caregivers likely will need to give ever increasing help for the duration of their loved one's journey. The right equipment can be significant in helping a loved one with safety while also helping to reduce the burden on the caregiver.

33
TRANSFER SKILLS TO KNOW

Caregivers will perform many transfers and having the right skills helps to minimize falls. Ask your physical therapist to educate you on the best way to transfer your loved one. They may have some specific techniques that will help you.

In the meantime, here are some tips that may be helpful. First and foremost...

** ALWAYS USE A GAIT BELT **

Your loved one may not like this, but it's about safety. Too many things can go wrong in a transfer so make sure you have a gait belt in place. Sometimes the difference between a disastrous fall is something as simple as this.

Sit to stand transfers.

The transfers that people struggle with most are the ones where their loved ones are sitting on a couch or recliner and have difficulty standing.

1) Have them practice scooting to the edge, leaning forward, and putting their "nose over their toes" prior to standing. This helps put their body weight in the best position to stand.

2) Then use their hands on the armrest as well as their legs to help themselves push up.

If they still struggle, you may want to consider getting a railing that goes on the couch or recliner. These will help your loved one have a firmer surface with which to stand.

It's also important how they sit back down. Elders tend to get into the habit of "plopping" into their chair due to decreased strength in their legs.

Encourage them and train them to do controlled sitting as if they ever do break something like a hip, the habit of plopping can be hard on the joints. Good habits pay long term dividends.

Surface-to surface-transfers

If your loved one has one leg stronger than the other, position the wheelchair that they are transferring to so that **they transfer to their strong side**. This will help reduce the likelihood of falls.

What about sliding boards? A sliding board is a board that goes under the loved one's bottom and then is also braced on the wheel-chair. Have them slide to their strong side.

Those with dementia often have difficulty using sliding boards as they can't figure out how to slide. But in the early stages for some they can be of help. Putting a pillow case under their bottom can help make the slide on the board a little bit easier. Also baby powder under the pillow case can help.

If you are using a wheelchair, always lock the brakes. ALWAYS. No exception.

Bathroom transfers

Sometimes when your loved one goes to sit, their aim can be off and they can wind up on the floor. Or worse, they can break something. Safety in bathroom transfers depend on the strength of their legs, the height of the toilet and their ability to balance.

It may be worth at some point considering getting a toilet safety frame and rail. This helps with controlling descent/ascent by giving them appropriate hand railings.

If your loved one has trouble standing up from the toilet, if the wall is close enough, you may want to install a grab bar. It just needs to be something more sturdy than the suction cup grab bar but something that can be nailed into the studs of the wall.

Caregivers will typically help their loved ones do thousands of transfers. Practice good habits to make sure you and your loved one can perform the safest transfer possible. Physical therapists can help train you how to do these effectively.

34
CAREGIVER DRIVEN MOBILITY

In the latter stages of dementia, mobility becomes more and more caregiver driven. Literally. Here are some pieces of equipment that are beneficial for later stages.

Wheelchairs

Wheelchairs are wonderful inventions and can be very helpful with older loved ones, even if they only need to take a rest while being pushed around. But wheelchairs need to be fit for the person.

A poorly fitting wheelchair can cause pressure ulcers, loss of circulation in the legs, etc... Most importantly there needs to be at least two fingers width on each side after the person is seated and four fingers of space between the end of the seat and the back of the knees. Physical therapy or occupational therapists can help with an accurate fitting and are highly recommended.

One factor in purchasing a wheelchair is also the weight of the wheelchair. There are lightweight, collapsible wheelchairs for those loved ones who weigh less and are mobile on the pavement. This helps the caregivers as they tend to lift the wheelchair in and out of the car often.

But, depending on the size of your loved one, they may need a standard or heavier wheelchair. And the terrain that they will cross. The heavier-duty wheelchairs do much better on gravel, grass, and variable terrains.

If you have Medicare Part B, they may help pay for it. And they also will help have it fitted to the person.

Hospital Beds

A bed can be an unexpected place of danger for loved ones in the mid to late stages. It is not hard to roll out of a bed and break a bone.

There are several options. You can purchase a railing that goes onto your current bed. You can also opt to add a mattress to the floor beside the bed in case your loved ones falls out.

However, at some point, standard beds become increasingly difficult to use and often less safe. A hospital bed may be a good option as it is easily raised and lowered helping the caregiver get their loved one in and out of bed. Additionally, the bed has railings on it preventing your loved one from rolling onto the floor at night.

There is often assistance with acquiring the beds from your Durable Medical Equipment department in your hospital. They typically do need a script from your doctor so consult your doctor regarding a bed. But insurance and/or Medicare can sometimes help supply these.

Lifts

A lift is something that may seem scary to use but they really are not as complicated as they look. With proper training from your physical therapist, a home lift can make a world of difference. A simple to use lift that is a possibility is a "Get-U-Up" lift. These come in manual hydraulic or fully electric.

One thing to consider is that if your area sometimes has electricity outages from storms, rolling blackouts, or other events, you might need to consider your options. A manual lift is not electricity dependent but it does take about 20-30 pumps on the handle to raise your loved one.

If a caregiver has bad shoulders, then an electric lift may be a better option. Go with the lift your physical therapist and/or doctor recommends and that is best fit for your loved one and you as the caregiving using the piece of equipment.

Yes, these things are pricey. But you can sometimes find used ones on social media marketplaces or in medical lending closets. Good options are out there.

A Hoyer lift is another common lift. These are full-body lifts and helpful with transferring your loved one from one place to another. These are made for fully dependent persons.

The challenge with these kinds of lifts is that getting the sling under your loved one can be a two-person or more job. Add to that they are not the best to use with bathroom needs.

The right medical equipment at the right time fitting in the right way can help you and your loved one tremendously. Caregivers literally perform thousands of transfers. It's not only about your loved one at this point, but about the best equipment for you also as the caregiver, minimizing injury to you.

35
WHEELCHAIR RAMP SIZING

W hen you are working with higher-level care, especially with caregiver-driven mobility, one thing that might need to be considered is adding a wheelchair ramp to your home. A physical or occupational therapist can help give you direction with this and there may even be financial assistance from the government to help install one (check with your OT/PT or doctor).

Here are some general guidelines.

<u>What are the appropriate measurements for a wheelchair ramp?</u>

The ratio of angle is 1:12. For every 1 inch of height, you need 12 inches of length. An easier way to think of it is for every 1 inch of height you need 1 foot of length. For example, if you have 15 inches of height from the ground to the top of your stairs, you will need 15 feet of length for the ramp. This is a gentle angle for wheelchairs and walkers. Making too steep a ramp is quite dangerous, especially in inclement weather.

<u>What handles do you need?</u>

Some people put 2x4 boards as the handles but this can be hard on your loved one's hands. They need to be rounded so that they can hold onto and grasp the railing with their fingers.

The height of the handles matter as well. Generally speaking you need the hand railing at around 32-36" in height and that railing to extend 1" beyond the ramp side boards.

What width do you need?

If it is a straight ramp, you will need a minimum width of approximately 36 inches between the hand railing. This is approximately 42 inches between the stabilizing boards.

If there is an area you need to turn around in you will need at least 60 inches of space. A 5'x5 landing often works best.

What about the flooring?

Make sure to have boards with small 1/4"spaces in between so that water can get through. When snow comes, you really do not want an icy slope.

Having said that, the boardwalk also needs to have anti-slip material attached. Anything sloped can quickly become a hazard during inclement weather. Always walk with your loved one with their gait belt secured around their waist and in your hands.

Adding a wheelchair ramp to your house may be an extra cost, but it can also serve to increase the value of your house. There is a large generation that is looking to retire and wheelchair accessibility is something more and more are having to consider.

But just make sure your ramp is not something that is dangerous. There are far too many that are so steep that loved ones cannot safely navigate the angle.

36

INSTRUCTIONS, CONCEPTUAL ABILITY AND VERBAL PROCESSING

When the brain takes a hit, so does its ability to conceptualize. When that happens the only thing a person sees in front of them is what is real. They can't necessarily imagine what is behind them or to the side.

For example, you might be performing a couch-to-chair transfer and instruct them to "move back towards the coach." For caregivers that means move their feet backward to where they can be seated. But for a loved one the words "move back" likely mean moving back to the original place they just came from prior to sitting on the couch.

They look where they were, and instead of moving back toward the couch, they move forward to where they have just been previously. It can be frustrating for a caregiver.

It comes down to learning a different language. "Left" and "right" do not make any more sense than "front" or "back" to a loved one in advanced stages of the disease. Sometimes you loved one will be able to think clearly and follow directions but sometimes they will not be able to do so.

Using different words can help. For example instead of saying "move back" you can say move "backward." Finding words that are more effective for them can help.

One tip with transfers is to use tape on the floor that is a strong contrast in color to your flooring. Put two "x's" where their feet need to go. As they approach the couch or chair, have them look at the "x's" and place their feet on the tape.

Keep directions short and simple. But the visual markers can be something that help in earlier stages. Be creative to the season that they are in.

It will take working with your loved one to find words that make sense to them. The different seasons that loved ones will go through in the process of the disease will be different so it is an ever-changing journey.

37
ALL ABOUT CARS

Your loved one will have a changing capacity to enter and exit a car. Skills to do so will typically be needed as loved ones have many doctor appointments.

Physical therapists can actually practice with you at your car making sure the appropriate safety techniques are in place. Please consult professional assistance but until then, here are some pointers.

Entry/Exit from a Car

If your loved one is in a walker, make sure they bring their walker close to the car door and not leave their walker several feet away and walk to the car. Establish good habits early.

Have them go all the way to the door, turn their walker to the side so it can still be used as a support as they move to the seated position first in the car. Then they can put in their legs.

If they are in a wheelchair and able to stand, bring them right up to the door and help them. (Make sure they have a gait belt on). One tool that might be helpful is a car handle assist. It can be placed where the door latches and provide a firm handle for your loved to hold onto.

It may come to the point at which you are unable to get them in and out of a car. If that is the case, oftentimes at the county level there is low-cost public transportation that has wheelchair lifts. They can help you go not only to doctor appointments but for community activities.

Just know they don't wait for you. You have to schedule pick-up times.

Inside the Car

You may think that your victory is won once you get your loved one inside the car. But that is not always the case.

Loved ones may not be clear in their thinking and try to open the door while going down the highway. Or they may be very active with their hands and try to reach for various items. If the window is open they may think they need to "clean" and will throw valuable things like their eyeglasses or shoes out the window (don't ask how this author knows).

Make sure your loved one is seat-belted into place and doors are locked. If you don't want things to go out the window, make sure they are rolled up.

If they tend to want to reach for everything, provide them with objects for their hands. Typical reachers/grabbers may or may not work depending on the level of their motor skill. Sometimes long kitchen tongs can help them to reach fallen items.

Managing the Lewy Lean While You Drive

The Lewy Lean is the heavy lean to one side. If it happens to be that their lean is to the left, it can affect your driving ability. One thing that can help in addition to seat belting them is a neck pillow. If their neck is hindered from falling all the way to the side, their lean is somewhat lessened, although not completely.

Some may try pillows but those are not necessarily advisable. If they slip away and int your seat they too can hinder driver visibility.

Typically caregivers will need to transport their loved ones often. Make sure to have measures in place to do this safely and effectively. Use a gait belt and the equipment needed for the season.

38
DURABLE MEDICAL EQUIPMENT (DME)

I t can be overwhelming to look at the equipment needed, the costs entailed and what equipment to get at what time. Do not stress as you will not need all the equipment all at once.

Talk to your doctor about what insurance or Medicare can cover for medical equipment. Surprisingly it can help with a lot more than most people realize. You must be enrolled in Medicare Part B though to receive these benefits.

Here is a list of common things that Medicare Part B Covers:

- Discounted protein drinks
- Blood sugar meters and test strips
- Canes
- Commode chairs
- Continuous passive motion machines and more
- Hospital beds
- Infusion pumps and supplies
- Nebulizers and medications
- Oxygen equipment and accessories

- Patient lifts
- Pressure reducing support surfaces
- Suction pumps
- Traction Equipment
- Walkers
- Wheelchairs and Scooters

Your doctors and DME suppliers must also be enrolled in Medicare. Ask a supplier if they participate in Medicare before you get any equipment. If suppliers are not enrolled in Medicare, there is no cap on what they can charge and it could get quite expensive.

What is your cost? After you meet the Medicare Part B Deductible, you will still pay 20% of the cost. But there are other factors involved depending on if you need to rent the equipment or buy it outright. If you have supplementary insurance they may also help with the costs.

If you need something in particular, it will take getting a script/prescription for that piece of medical equipment from your primary care provider. Consult them and let them know of your present needs.

Equipment can be a lot, but it is necessary. Look for various outlets that can help like medical lending closets. Consult your doctor to see if they know of charities that can also assist. Explore social media marketplaces. If you go with used equipment, you need to know that it is safe and in good working order. Consult your physical therapist for help.

HOSPITAL STAYS & MEDICAL CARE

39
MEDICAL ITEMS FOR YOUR REFRIGERATOR LIST

M edical incidents cannot be predicted, they just happen. Whether it is a fall, an episode of something unexpected, or any other medical incident, readiness helps reduce stress. Also the main caregiver might not be the one home with your loved one at the time. Therefore it is good to have a "refrigerator list." These will also serve for routine doctor appointments.

By putting medical information on the refrigerator, it becomes quickly accessible to anyone who needs to use it in an emergency. If they are on top of the refrigerator as opposed to a magnet clip, make sure everyone knows about the papers and where they are at.

Things you will need:

1) <u>Updated Medication List</u> - This needs to be updated whenever there is a medical change. But keep a list of all medications, the dosages (milligrams) and how often they take the pills. On that page, it also needs to include your loved one's name and birthdate. Also include emergency contact information for you, the caregiver(s).

2) <u>A list of contraindications</u> for the type of dementia your loved one has printed from a respectable dementia website.

This is especially true with Lewy Body Dementia as it is unique to the other dementias. Make sure to include "Behavior Drugs to Avoid" and "Other Drugs to Avoid" including Haldol/Halperidol that can be printed from the LBDA.org website.

Print any Medical Alert Wallet Card if it is available on the respective websites. Have it ready to give to medical staff when needed with emergencies or routine doctor appointments.

Lewy Body Dementia – <u>www.LBDA.ORG</u>

Parkinson's Disease – <u>www.Parkinson.org</u>

Alzheimer's – <u>www.Medicalert.com</u>

Other forms of dementia – <u>www.alzstore.com</u>

DIY Medical Alert Card - https://amzn.to/3rucqH2

3) <u>DNR paperwork (Do not Resuscitate)</u> - If your loved one does not want to be resuscitated in case of a medical crisis, make sure that this paperwork is available to give to the hospital.

Have all these items ready to go before a medical incident. Place them in a public, visible way for you and also other family members. The refrigerator is a great place for these.

This kind of information will also be needed when you go for a routine doctor's visit so it is good to have multiple copies. Check out the bonuses section in this book to get an Emergency Planner "What If" Printable. This will help you stay organized.

Unexpected events happen. But by being prepared, you reduce the stress and increase safety measures for your loved one.

40

DEALING WITH FALLS

F alls are very real and unfortunately not uncommon with those who have dementia. Stability and balance are major factors. You can do everything to keep your loved one safe and have every piece of equipment you can think of and still it's possible for your loved one to have a fall.

Take falls seriously. If they have hit their head they may need to have their head medically examined to make sure no stroke or bleeds in the brain are occurring from the fall.

If they are complaining of hip pain, it is very possible that they might have broken a hip. The cardinal signs of a hip fracture are that the leg rotates outwards, the knee bends out, the leg seems to shorten, and there are intermittent unbearable spasms of pain.

Call the ambulance. Even if you do not see these signs, if your loved has fallen and is in pain of any kind, call the ambulance. Do not risk an untreated injury.

Here are some important tips:

1) Do not move your loved one. Make them comfortable with blankets and pillows and let them know that help is on the way.

2) While you are waiting for the ambulance, make sure you have a list of medications and their dosages. Use "the Refrigerator List." The ambulance crew will ask for these upon arrival.

3) Decide which hospital you would like to take your loved one.

4) Determine the best way for the ambulance to enter your house with a stretcher. Then when the ambulance arrives direct them accordingly.

5) When they arrive let them know your loved one has dementia. Do this discreetly as if your loved one hears it may increase their agitation because of embarrassment.

Oftentimes your loved one will be checked over and given some pain medicine prior to loading them up in the ambulance. If the ambulance crew is willing, sometimes you can ride with them.

Although it can be best just to go in your own car. Pack some overnight clothes, basic toiletries, and a book as the process can be hours/days long. Also take your loved one's medications, although at the hospital they may pause these depending on the doctor.

Typical Protocol for US Residents:

Typically upon arrival to the hospital, they will take some x-rays after your loved in check in. If there is no stroke or other abnormalities, your loved one will be sent home.

If it is a hip break, they will keep your loved one on pain medication and then schedule surgery. Surgery isn't necessarily right away as surgeons have a line-up of cases. It oftentimes takes place in the middle of the night or the next day. Sometimes it can even take several days.

Should you have someone stay with your loved one?

Not all hospitals will let you stay with your loved one. Some will. Talk to the head of nursing. Explain to them that your loved one has dementia and you would like to stay with them to minimize issues for your loved one and call for help if needed.

It is the author's opinion that if it all possible and permitted by the nursing staff, you should stay with them. It helps your loved one navigate a confusing scenario as well as help keep them safe.

If your loved one has surgery, they may be in the hospital for a week or more depending on their condition.

Prior to Surgery

Know that recent studies are showing that general anesthesia can be hard on the brain with certain types of dementia, again most often with Lewy Body Dementia. Sometimes you have no choice in the matter as surgery is better than not having it.

If Lewy Body Dementia is the diagnoses of your loved one, check with the lbda.org association for recommendations. Also talk with your anesthesiologist about possible alternatives that they would recommend.

Post Surgery

It is not uncommon for those with dementia to have increased delusions during extended hospital stays. There are a number of factors for this.

At the same time the doctors may be monitoring for strokes and such if delusions increase. Let them do their work.

Lengthy hospital stays can also cause "hospital psychosis." This is where delusions and hallucinations significantly increase. Talk to your doctor about management strategies.

41

KNOWING ABOUT MEDICARE FOR HOSPITAL STAYS (FOR US CITIZENS)

Medicare is the US national health service for American citizens. It is mainly for those who are over 65 and for younger people with notable disabilities. At 65 if you want Medicare you will need to enroll your loved one (which is highly recommended). You can do so at Medicare.gov.

There are several parts to Medicare benefits:

- Medicare Part A (Hospital Insurance) – Part A covers inpatient hospital stays, care in a skilled nursing facility, hospice care, and some home health care.

- Medicare Part B (Medical Insurance)- Part B covers certain doctor services, outpatient care, medical supplies, and preventive services.

- Medicare Part D (prescription drug coverage) – Helps cover the cost of prescription drugs (including many recommended shots or vaccines).

If your loved one has a hospital stay or is in a nursing rehabilitation unit, at present with Medicare Part A the therapists are required to provide 720 minutes (12 hours) of therapy per week between 2 to 3 of the disciplines of physical, occupational, and speech therapy. The patient and the family can decide based on need whether they want 2 or 3 of the disciplines. The most common ones are physical therapy and occupational therapy.

At present anything less than those 720 minutes and the facility will not get reimbursed at all from Medicare. So there is pressure on the therapists to get the full 720 minutes in for the week.

Anything over the 720 minutes and the facility does not get any extra reimbursement. Again, it is hard on the facility as it means they gave free care while paying their staff. Because of this, therapies are trying their best to get a minimum of 720 minutes in per week and not much over.

Why is this important to you? There is a reason that when a therapist comes into a room and a patient only wants to do 10 minutes of therapy that the therapist will give exhortation to go longer. The therapists need to get their minutes in for that week. If you only go 10 minutes one day, you will need to do more minutes the next day to ensure the 720 total minutes per week is reached among the cumulative disciplines. It is a careful tightrope that the therapists walk.

As for Part B it is not such a big issue. Part B of Medicare has no specific minute guideline so it is driven by what is ideal for the patient.

Understanding Medicare services for therapy is helpful so next time you are in the hospital with your loved and they need rehab care, you will better understand the therapist's role. They want your very best but they too are under constraints.

If you have questions there typically is someone who is a caseworker that can help you navigate the intricacies. If they are not available you can talk with your medical professionals who can direct you to a person who can help.

42
UNDERSTAND THE DIFFERENT THERAPIES

Your loved one goes to the hospital for some reason and at discharge, they ask if you want home health, physical therapy, occupational therapy, speech and/or speech therapy. The truth is many are just guessing at what those therapies are and how they relate to your loved one. Here is a summary:

Home health – Home health is made up of nursing staff who come to regularly check up on your loved one after a hospital stay or medical event. This is highly recommended to monitor your loved one's health.

Physical Therapy (PT)--Physical Therapy often focuses on restoring the large muscle groups after an injury, surgery or a medical event. In a skilled nursing facility in particular, the difference between occupational therapy vs physical therapy is that physical therapy will deal primarily with the lower extremities (legs) while occupational therapy will focus more on the upper extremities (arms and hands).

Occupational Therapy (OT)–Occupational Therapy focuses on everyday functional skills such as taking a shower, dressing, sorting pills, etc... They also help with adaptive equipment for functionality in the home. Working with fine motors skills in the hands is their specialty. They also help strengthen shoulders and arms.

They may use some exercise equipment but most of OT will concentrate on using regular household items. Additionally, their focus often rests on the use of the hands, arms and fingers. The fine motor skills are a main focus of occupational therapy.

Speech Therapy (ST) – Speech therapy is not solely focused on talking, although this is often the case in working with younger people. For the geriatric population, their main focus is on helping with swallowing and feeding issues.

Considering that swallowing can become difficult in later stages, this resource may be one you need. Speech therapy can also work with alternative forms of communication when speech is impaired.

When your loved one is discharged from the hospital or sometimes even just from medical appointments, the doctor may ask you if you would like one or more of these therapies. It is up to you and is dependent on the condition for which they are being treated and for what they need at the time. You can choose all the therapies or only a few.

43
AQUATIC THERAPY

Aquatic therapy is an amazing form of therapy for loved ones, especially in the earlier and middle stages of dementia. Although at the same you have to be highly cautious and take their abilities and capabilities on an individual basis.

1) Gauge the diagnosis and the current status of your loved one to know if aquatic therapy is a good fit. Check with your doctor.

2) Call the pool and make sure a lifeguard is on duty. If not, keep searching for one that does have a lifeguard available.

If it is a good fit, there are many good things with water. Water can take the weight off of the joints and make it easier to move. If a person wobbles while walking, the water can catch their fall. By taking away some of the fear of falling there can be greater liberty of movement.

You can even request professional aquatic therapy with physical therapy. Sometimes it can be prescribed by your doctor if the conditions are right.

Initially just start with water acclimation. Sometimes even if someone has spent their whole life in water, they may need time to adjust. Just sitting in knee or chest-deep water at the edge of the pool can accomplish this. It may take several weeks or more depending on your loved one.

This can then progress to supervised water walking. It can also help strengthen their leg muscles and core which is valuable for mobility activities when on land. Confidence can be slowly gained as movement in the water progresses at the rate of your loved one's comfort level and ability.

You can progress from there to doing simple exercises and leg and arm movements. Full-on swimming is not suggested without a caregiver and/or lifeguard in the water standing beside them. Facilities can sometimes offer classes that can help make social connections for your loved one.

Water also has a side benefit for the caregivers. When you are working with an older loved one, the caregiver's own physical activity is often minimal. By helping a loved one it can also improve the health of the caregiver as you also move in the water.

Check into facilities near you. Here are some questions to ask:

1) Do you have a ramp into and out of your pool?

2) Do you have a lift that is handicap accessible with trained staff to operate?

3) Are there classes available that are predominantly elderly (or for your loved one's needs)?

4) What is the cost of a day pass?

5) Do you have a lifeguard on duty at all times?

Aquatic therapy is one of the best ways to help your loved one preserve some of their strength. Go slowly as they may need to acclimate to being in the water after being out for a while.

- Make sure you or someone with you with is a competent swimmer in case there are problems.

- Never leave your loved one alone.

- Swim in shallow water

- Use floatation devices.

- Swim with a gait belt on for quick ability to hold them up if needed

- Make sure a lifeguard is on duty

Here are some ways in which a loved one is NOT a good fit:

- Do not swim if your loved one has advanced stages of dementia

- If your loved one has open wounds, they should not for any reason be in a public water situation

- If they have bowel or bladder incontinence, aquatic therapy may not be a good fit

- If they have had a lifelong fear of water and do not know how to swim, it isn't a good time to start

Know your loved one. Adjust according to their needs. It's something that can be a really good option under the right circumstances.

44

IMPORTANT PHARMACEUTICAL FACTORS

U nderstanding dementia is never more important than when it comes to pharmaceuticals. Things like Lewy Body dementia have a very separate pathology from Parkinson's and Alzheimer's and as such have different drug intolerances.

What can you do?

1) Be Informed – Know and understand as much about your loved one's form of dementia as you can.

2) Look for a doctor, neurologist, or specialist who has skills with dementia. Or at least one who is open to study and learn more about your loved one's form of dementia.

3) Know your treatment options. Find medical professionals who will work with you and your loved for the best desired outcomes.

4) Understand that most primary care physicians are typically not specialists but rather generalists. They deal with countless conditions and each disease has countless indications and contraindications, or medicines that are beneficial and not recommended.

Print off any medical card from an official website pertaining to your loved one's form of dementia.

Pharmaceutical Observations for Medicines They Do Take

Working with pharmaceutical interventions is a tricky process. Every person is different. What works great for one person does not work well for another person. Just because a medication is prescribed does not mean that it is the ideal fit for your loved one.

Observe your loved one.

- Is the medication helping?
- Are you seeing adverse responses?
- Are they stumbling more?
- Is there an increase of confusion?

If there are significant adverse changes, call your doctor. They too need to know. Pharmacology isn't an exact science as every person is so unique. Communicate well.

Naturopathic or Not?

Sometimes after trying traditional pharmaceutical meds and not seeing the results that are wanted, some people turn to naturopathic support. Make sure if you go this route, you consult someone who is highly trained. If your naturopath has a doctorate in naturopathic medicine it is preferred.

Go to their business and check it out. Make sure to find a store with high standards of excellence and not a closet, hobbyist corner shop. Quality matters.

Additionally, stay connected with your traditional primary care provider. There can be interactions between medicines and supplements. Good communication is necessary for the best and safest results for your loved one.

45

CHOKING MATTERS

As dementia progresses, your loved one will have a harder time chewing and swallowing liquids. So much so that many with dementia pass away from pneumonia as a result of aspirating food or liquid.

You must monitor their ability to swallow. Especially in later stages. Here are some ways you can help them.

1) Consult a speech therapist. Their job is not just about talking but about all things with the mouth. They can help give you and your loved one strategies for swallowing.

2) Use thickened liquids such as fruit smoothies or commercial thickeners. If it is a bit thicker your loved one will be able to swallow liquids easier.

3) Cook appropriately. Big, chewy chunks of steak are probably not going to be ideal in mid to later stages. Use hamburger or other proteins that are soft. Cut any meat up in very small pieces. Use meats like chicken over tougher meats like steak. Learn to cook differently with foods like rice and beans or various kinds of pasta.

4) Assist them with sitting upright. This is not as easy as it sounds when the Lewy lean is strong. Add pillows to their wheelchair and use a neck pillow to help keep their head in a more neutral position.

5) Make sure they drink before meals and during the meal to keep their mouths wet.

6) Still make food flavorful. They will need the motivation to eat healthy and eat well. The better it tastes for them, the more motivation. In fact, sometimes taste can be one of their last remaining pleasures in the end stages.

The farther along in the journey of the disease, the more choking becomes a very real matter to attend to by the caregiver. Make sure you do what you can to assist your loved one with food and liquids that are more suited to their stage of living.

46

FACILITATING TOOTH AND NAIL CARE

D aily care is something we all do without even thinking about it. But it is not something that your loved one can do on their own.

Tooth Care

Dental care is an important part of maintaining your loved one's health as bacteria can get into the bloodstream through poor dental hygiene. At the same time, it can be challenging for both loved ones and/or caregivers to do a good job of proper tooth and gum maintenance for the loved one. Here are some tips:

1) Continue with regular cleanings every 6 months if possible. This is also important as your dentist can see if any problems are forming such as abscesses, infections, or other areas of concern.

2) Use mouthwash regularly to help them with bacteria, especially at night. It's not just about bad breath, it's about bacteria reduction.

3) If they have trouble with them leaning far enough over the sink to rinse out their mouth, have them sit, brush their teeth and rinse

their mouth into a small plastic tub. It can reduce stress for both your loved one and you as the caregiver.

4) Use only a small bit of toothpaste as it will do the trick without over-frothing in the mouth.

5) Be aware of posture to avoid choking and aspiration. This will matter when they get to the point of the Lewy Lean. Try to put them upright and support them as best as possible.

Your loved one may or may not be eager to brush their teeth. The time eventually comes when you will need to help them completely. But until then there are some things you can do.

1) Brush your teeth with them. Make it fun. This is a form of mirroring.

2) Use a timer to make sure brushing goes long enough. Make the final sound a celebratory one and not an alarm-sounding timer.

3) Coach them but do not correct them in a way that appears scolding. They may need directions and encouragement for the processes.

Dental hygiene is often overlooked as there are so many other factors that loved ones and caregivers are dealing with. But issues with the gums in particular can cause other health issues that can be avoided.

Hand and Nail Care

Another form of hygiene is their hands and fingernails. Because of their loss of fine motor skills, your loved can often acquire some not-so-pleasant dark matter stuck underneath their fingernails after using the bathroom.

First of all, help them wash their hands. Make it fun, rubbing their hands under warm water. Soap their hands up well and wash away.

Second, help them keep their nails trimmed and clean. Smaller-sized nails mean less gunk underneath. If it gets too out of control, you can take them in for a manicure and/or pedicure.

If your loved one is in a hospital, nursing staff typically will not take care of their nails. The reason is if they cause a bleed and it gets infected, they are afraid of lawsuits. In a hospital situation, only podiatrists or family can manage nails. So if your loved one has a prolonged stay in the hospital, you can ask for a podiatrist or take care of what you need.

47

COMMON COMMUNITY RESOURCES (US CITIZENS)

You cannot know what you don't know, but there are oftentimes more resources out there than we realize that are ready to help you take care of your loved one. Ask your doctor, your therapists, and others what resources they know that help assist in the journey. Here are some important resources:

1) <u>Area Council on Aging Respite Care</u> — Some states can help on the caregiving journey. It's not uncommon if the circumstances are right for the state to pay for on average of 12-16 hours of respite care a month. They typically are contracted out with professionals and those hours can be divided in the month how it is best seen fit. Contact your local agency and see what they all have to offer.

2) <u>Post-Hospitalization Bath Aides</u> - After a hospitalization, talk with your caseworker about getting a bath aide. Sometimes they will pay for bath aides to come help with showers 1-2x per week for on average 6 months after hospitalization. If your loved one is open to this, it can be help reduce the burden of care on the caregivers.

3) <u>Medical Equipment Lending Closets</u> - Surprisingly there are often medical equipment lending closets in your area. And if they are not in your area, they sometimes can deliver equipment to your door. Usually there is a very small fee and the time frame of borrowing is around 6 months, but these can be great ways to cut down on equipment costs.

4) <u>Hospice</u> - When a loved one looks to be about 6 months or so from passing away, hospice can sometimes come in and help with care, costs, pain management, and more.

If you want to check on specific resources for your area, if you are a US citizen type in your zip code at https://eldercare.acl.gov. They provide a great list of organizations and services that could be a huge benefit for you and your loved one.

CAREGIVER TIPS

48

THE PURPOSE OF YOUR HOUSE

Here's an inconvenient truth. If you choose to keep your loved one at home, it will get dinged up. Corners will get scuffed from wheelchairs and walkers, holes might need to be put in the walls for railings, grab bars may need to be installed in the shower, your furniture might suffer from episodes of incontinence, and your loved one pulling hard on the furniture.

It's like having a child again. No one who has children has a house that has survived unscathed from their children. And now the roles are reversed. Your house typically will not make it undamaged by taking care of your loved ones.

It is helpful on an emotional level for you as the caregiver to decide early on what purpose the house you have serves. Are you meant to serve the house or is the house meant to serve your needs? Same with your car. It too can get dirty and marked up.

If you are regularly frustrated when walls get marked by walkers or wheelchairs, then you will be in a place of constant frustration and aggravation because it will continue. But if you accept this as a reality, it will become the least of your concerns in your journey.

There are things you can do.

- Put carpet barriers on corners.

- Put out used furniture that is not concerning if damaged.

- Put aside special items that would be hard on you if they were broken.

These things may seem small. But sometimes they are not. They can even cause familial stress. Settle in your minds that adaptation of your house and loved one is par for the course. Do your best to minimize damage, but at the same time, it is good to be realistic. Adjust accordingly. Both practically and emotionally.

It helps to remember that when the time is right that many things can be fixed. It is a small price to pay for love and it is one that our loved one paid for us when we were young and dependent.

49
MANAGING THOUGHTS AND FEELINGS

C aregiving can have some great moments, but also some really low moments. This is especially true if the journey goes on for more than a couple of years. So many sacrifices are made and there is no end date in sight. You don't know how to plan or live your own life and you don't even know if it is even possible.

Attitude. Is. Everything.

If you are a naturally optimistic person and nothing phases you, then head on to the next chapter. For the rest of humanity, a positive and good attitude can be difficult at times. Especially when you are exhausted, frustrated, and have no idea how it is going to work out financially and practically.

Because of the intensity of the season though, if you allow even the smallest of negative thoughts, you will be in tears, anger, and frustration within mere seconds. In lesser seasons, this likely would not happen. But the pressure of caregiving can take you down that road lightning fast.

Guard. Your. Thoughts.

You will miss them when they are gone. So be careful about what you are thinking about. Here are some dangerous thoughts to avoid:

- Self-pity
- Comparison to others' situations
- Excessive complaining about your circumstances in your own thoughts or to others

These can very easily come into our minds and if we are not diligent, we will fall into frustration and anger more quickly than we realize. It then spills over into our relationship with our loved one and our relationships with those around us.

Here are some things to consider:

1) Understand that we are on this earth to love one another.

That is one of our highest purposes in life. You may want to travel, fulfill desires and dreams, and do other things, but if you love well, you have done life well. Everything we do is about loving one another.

At the end of the day love, when given a chance, will also change you. Many selfish tendencies are stripped down and exposed. We are confronted with our own humanity. It is a gift to actually get to see and deal with these and grow from them.

2) By caring for our loved ones, we are training our family and others how to love us when the time comes.

Many of us do not dream of one day ending up in a nursing home, especially in this day and age. By showing love to our elders, we are teaching children and grandchildren how to take care of us. Through kindness. Care. And keeping loved ones home as long as possible.

3) You get to help redefine the narrative.

One of the biggest problems, at least in a lot of Western culture, is that we have set up a paradigm of how life should go. It is often assumed that a person grows up,

graduates, goes to college, gets married, has kids, and then retires and travels.

What is left out of this equation is caring for elderly parents and staying at home with them. And then when their care comes up, and they cannot travel and do whatever, people can become bitter.

We need to shift the paradigm to working, retiring, traveling a short time, and taking care of family as long as necessary. That is not in our paradigm... yet. You help change that by caring for your loved one.

In many other cultures in the world, they don't believe in nursing homes. The whole family system, the aunts, cousins, brothers and sisters, take care of their elders and it is considered a joy and privilege. It's just what you do.

This is a healthy way of care and very life-giving. Who knows that we might not one day be forced to return to his model given world circumstances?

There are exceptions as some people just cannot care for their loved ones at home as it becomes too much. This is Ok. We are all in different situations. But by you loving your family at home as long as possible, you help redefine the national story of caregiving.

Yes, caregiving has many costs involved. Most will never know the cost you will pay. Or how deep it cuts. But the sacrifice is worth it. Love is worth it.

Your parents likely took care, sacrificing for you for many years when you were young. This is a way we can give back. .

50

SETTING BOUNDARIES FOR PEOPLE

As caregivers, emotional energy is in short supply. At the same time, there are many friends who love us and want to help. Some of them help in good ways, and others try but just don't understand what way is best.

1) <u>From the beginning, you will need to set boundaries with people</u>. If there is interference with health care decisions or someone demonstrating lack of appropriate boundaries, gently and lovingly draw the line. If you do not do so early you will pay a high price for it later. Sometimes you will have to get firm if gentleness hasn't worked after repeated efforts of communication.

2) <u>Do not assume that your best friend or the friend of the family is the ideal source of help</u>. Sometimes they are and sometimes they are not. Best friends may feel more free to interfere with healthcare decisions. Know your friends. If they are emotionally healthy friends, they will respect the family when you need some space. Be wise. Also be careful not to rely on your best friends too much in a way that they feel burnt by your relationship. This too can be troublesome.

3) <u>For those who want to help, oftentimes they just need practical direction</u>. Help them help you if that is the case by communicating with them what you do need and do not need. Make a list of what things people can do that actually would be a blessing for you.

4) <u>Recognize that some friends will not get the same amount of time as before</u>. It is not intentional, it is necessary for survival. Your friend probably will not fully understand but energy for the long haul is essential. Communicate with them and let them know you still value them, but you are in a season to commit to your loved one

Dealing with those outside of the family can be an unexpected challenge. People do not understand why you can't just take off for the weekend and go have some fun. Why you don't just get away more and "take care of yourself." But caregiving isn't like raising a child. There are many other factors to consider.

The people in your life can be well-intentioned, but even the very best of your friends do not understand the level of commitment it takes as a dementia caregiver. But know that there are thousands of other caregivers out there just like you going through similar struggles. You are hidden, but you are not alone.

51
LOVING ON EMPTY -
CAREGIVER FATIGUE

C aregiver exhaustion can be extreme. It not only comes from the physical and emotional demands of being a caregiver, but also comes from navigating a mysterious disease with family that may or may not be of assistance. All of these typically come unexpectedly when the caregiver was plunged into the world of dementia.

What Can You Realistically Do?

1) Take advantage of respite care services. Your local Area Council on Aging may be able to point you to respite care services that your state will pay for to help you.

2) You may need to consider Adult Day Care services if you are able to afford it in order to get a break.

3) Call in family members for help.

4) When your loved one sleeps, try to get sleep yourself. Sleep deprivation can affect every hour of your life. If things do not get done around the house, it is Ok. Your life will not be perfect in this season.

5) Stay connected with friends, even if it is just by phone.

6) Draw boundaries with those who might try to interfere or bring toxicity into the caregiving situation. You don't need the added stress.

7) Think of tasks that can be done more efficiently. Things such as cooking meals ahead of time or having groceries delivered to your home.

8) Get outside often in the fresh air and sunshine. It will help not only you but your loved one as well.

9) Find activities you can do with your loved one that are enjoyable to you. They may not always end well based on your loved one's emotional status, but things will sometimes turn out better than planned and you will have a good time together. Make memories.

The fatigue of caregiving will vary in intensity depending on the stage your loved one is in. Make sure you do what you can to give yourself grace.

52

ONE OF THE MOST
IMPORTANT CAREGIVER TIPS

Caregiving is not like what most of us expect. Many things do not unfold as we hoped or planned. Hard things occur:

- Family members that you thought would help may or may not be of assistance

- Unexpected people say harsh things if you take care of your loved one at home and do not put them into a nursing facility

- People you've known your whole try to intervene in ways you just cannot believe

- Medical staff may or may not be helpful

- Marital partners may or may not be supportive

- How someone lives, dies, and is buried is fought over

- And then there's the finances and inheritance and the sale of the house.

Worse is that if you are an at-home caregiver, there's a good chance that you are empty on so many levels—physically, emotionally, spiritually, and mentally. You may be experiencing exhaustion so far beyond what is visible in your face but is felt deeply in your soul. Your finances may be hovering at near possibility, your emotions frazzled, and your frustration level with all things can be intense. In better times of life, you may be able to process and respond to others' behaviors more reasonably.

That might not be that season.

Understand that generally speaking people do not get it. They just don't. Your circumstances are unique. And how you thought others would respond is not how they actually respond. Therefore we must grow in our ability to forgive.

Forgiveness is a practice. It is a process. It is a journey. When you forgive you have to keep on forgiving.

The problem is if we do not forgive we can become bitter, Bitterness of the soul makes it exponential harder to care for our loved one. It can lead to a resentment that spreads to the many, poisoning our hearts and sapping our strength.

Yes, relationships change. Some relationships can continue. Some cannot.

But we must all work on forgiving one another in love.

53
CHALLENGING FAMILY ISSUES

In your mind, you probably assume other immediate members of the family will help out equally. Unfortunately, that is not the case more often than not. It is more common that one person or household takes on the main responsibility and the help of others is minimal. This can be crushing. Not just from the work load but from the confusion of why others are not helping.

The anger and resentment that a caregiver can go through can cost not only familial relationships but also the quality of their own lives and hearts. Bitterness is a destructive force.

If you are in this situation, is there anything you can do?

1) Trying having a sit-down conversation and not just conversations in passing, letting them know the reality of your need and the kind of help you would appreciate. State your feelings and needs without accusation.

2) There may be a point where no matter how much you communicate, they still will do nothing to help. Here's an unpleasant reality.

You may just have to accept this and move on, not allowing the anger to change you.

3) If there is a continuous refusal to help, you might need to completely release any sense of expectation of assistance. Doing so will help you release your frustration.

4) Forgive. Forgive. Forgive.

Here's another reality. Some family may want to be involved but may be in conflict of how things best should be done. This isn't easy either. Do your best to communicate calmly and clearly.

The truth is walking this through with family is more times than not a hard, testing process. Everyone sees their role and responsibility differently. Guard your heart. Work towards finishing with your relationships intact.

54

SOCIAL MEDIA GROUPS - ARE THEY WORTH IT?

Dementia caregiver Facebook groups are usually the first place you go to when you learn of the diagnosis. You are at your wits end. You are often sleep-deprived, not sure who to believe in the medical world, and are hungry for help and community.

At first the Facebook forums seem like a lifeline. What you find are people who understand you and get your situation. Others don't understand but they do. You feel like you have found a handhold in the unsteady world of caregiving.

They are wonderful and lifesaver in the beginning. But after awhile you begin to realize something.

Many of the caregiver groups you joined are increasingly negative. Critical. And even in an internet group, you discover there is a power hierarchy.

Some things are allowed to say and some are not. Mention the wrong thing and you encounter piranhas. Say the right thing and you are a hero.

You begin to have mixed feelings. Do I stay with it and deal with the negativity in exchange for the knowledge and understanding I'm receiving? Or do I ditch it for the cause of staying filled with hope?

What are the advantages?

- You are with people who understand

- You meet a few good people who do not feel the need to rant on all occasions

- You do learn some helpful tips

What were the disadvantages?

- Most caregiver Facebook groups are heavy, despairing, and full of rants

- The disease of dementia becomes the center of your thoughts and world

- It becomes emotionally toxic after a season and if you are not careful, you will begin to go to a place of increased self-pity.

What are some possibilities to counter this?

- Start your own group and set the boundaries from the beginning of what you will or will not discuss and accept.

- Join a group for a short season to garner information that you need for your specific diagnosis and then leave.

In general, for mental health Facebook groups or other social media groups may only be advisable for a short amount of time. If a group is critical even in small percentages, the negativity and despair will rub off on you making the long haul of caregiving increasingly difficult.

Your perspective and heart matter too much to be around one more source of negativity. Learn what you can. Make some connections.

Ultimately it is your choice. Just make sure to find the places and groups that are life-giving.

55
SHOULD YOU TELL YOUR LOVED ONE ABOUT DIFFICULT EVENTS?

If someone passes away, should you tell your loved one? What about if the family pet dies? Or a friend or relative? At what point do you tell your loved one difficult things that have happened and at what point do you not?

This can be controversial, even more so among family members. At the end of the day the decision is best in the hands of the primary caregiver.

Generally speaking though, your loved one also wants to know and grieve their losses. It is Ok for them to mourn. It is normal.

Depending on the stage they are in, they probably will not remember one day to the next of a sad event that has happened. But if they do remember, how do you handle it?

After you've told them the first time, if they continue to ask over and over again, then it becomes a point where you do need to practice discretion. If they are reminded repeatedly that someone or something like a pet has died, for them it is like experiencing it for the first time, again.

From this point it may be worth telling them their pet is "in a good place" or "outside" (which is normally true considering a pet's burial), or something else that may be a bit more comforting.

Of course every person's temperament and situation is very different. How you choose to handle tough situations is fully at your discretion. You know your loved one best.

Know their stage of cognition. These things are something to talk about and consider with your family members when an event happens so you can be in one accord of how to handle hard situations.

56

THE STRANGEST, GREAT ADVICE

No joke, it sounds unkind. Nonsensical. And just... strange. But in the long run it can be some of the best advice.

"Do not make dementia the focus of your life.
Just talk about it as needed. That's it."

How could this be good advice? It sounds... cold. Uncaring. Calloused. But there's a nugget of truth hidden in that suggestion.

When someone has dementia, it is very easy to fall into the trap that dementia and caregiving take over your world. This doesn't have to be the case. When you can talk about dementia and caregiving needs on an as-needed basis and not make it at the center of most discussions, you can begin to enjoy life again. Dementia does not define your household. You do.

It was some of the best advice the author was given. Do not let dementia be the center. Still live life. Dementia and caregiving may try to dominate every aspect of your thoughts and life. But it doesn't have to be that way if you don't let it.

57
WILL THEY STILL KNOW ME?

One of the hard things for caregivers to contemplate is the question if your loved one will forget who you are as their family. And the answer is both a "yes" and "no."

Because of how the brain is affected by dementia, it is generally speaking only a matter of time before your loved one will forget names and how a person is connected to them such as if they are a son, daughter, spouse, friend, etc.... They may even ask, "Who are you?"

BUT it is the author's experience that they still do have a knowledge of who you are. Loved ones can still know and be comforted by your presence and know your voice.

They recognize you are familiar and loved, but they just can't remember your name or how they are related to you. It is not that they don't want to, but it's that part of the brain that remembers details that is affected.

Granted when they are in a bout of paranoia, that may not temporarily to be the case. But when the paranoia episode passes, their sense of familiarity will still be there.

Be encouraged though. It isn't that they have forgotten you. Your presence and your voice matter. You are what is familiar and loved, just minus the details that their brain can't quite figure out.

58

HAVE FUN TOGETHER

A diagnosis of dementia in a loved one should not be the end to living life. Neither for you or for them. Yes, it can be hard. But it isn't hard all the time.

The caregiving season is not just about caring for them to the end of their life, but also about creating good memories together. There are still many things you can do with them throughout their journey:

- Go on a walk/push their wheelchair together in the park while looking at lakes and beautiful flowers

- Go out to a favorite restaurant, even if you have to feed them

- Go shopping or stroll through the mall on a hot summer's day

- Go to a park and have a cookout with family

- Attend youth sporting events and social occasions

- Travel and go on vacations together

- Discover new areas of interest that are wheelchair accessible

Do things that you both enjoy together so that it can be beneficial to you as well. Get outside into the fresh air and sunshine. It is good for the body and soul of everyone.

Yes, things will go wrong. There will be days that outings will be frustrating. But in the end, it is worth it both to you and your loved one. Even in illness life moves on. Move on together.

Some of the best memories you can make with your loved one are during the caregiving years. It is also some of your final years to do so.

59
STORING UP MEMORIES

Your loved one's passing may come soon or it might happen a decade or more later. One never knows. It is good to not just make memories but also to store them for later recall.

Record Their Voice

One of the things commonly missed after a loved one passes away is their voice. This can be especially true at birthdays, Christmas or special events.

Take the time now to record them singing "Happy Birthday" or "We Wish you a Merry Christmas." Record any song that connects to a special memory. These can be played for years to come and be a comfort in the healing process.

Take the Picture

Caregivers typically do not look their best. They are often tired and have a lot on their mind. Take the picture anyway.

Take photos of your loved one and take pictures of you with your loved one. Get professional family photos. These may be the very last pictures of your loved one and these memories will become treasures for generations to come.

<u>Record Their Stories</u>

If your loved one is sufficiently cognizant, on the good days have them tell you different stories about their lives, and your life and beginnings as well. Preserve the important events.

Record them in audio and/or also record them by writing them down. The stories are treasures for years to come.

Your story and your history are not just for you but your children, nieces and nephews and descendants. The generations need this family story as part of growing in their identity.

60

FINDING PURPOSE IN YOUR OWN LIFE

Caregiving is an unknown journey that is full of twists and turns. A caregiver has no idea the length of time they will need to be caregivers, how intense the caregiving season will be, or how much they will need to handle versus how much other family will help.

The caregiving season is about sacrifice. Sacrifice is about giving up something you love for something you love even more. In this case, it is your loved one.

The reality is that a caregiver's own hopes, dreams, and ambitions at times are set aside, and for good reason. There are times when you cannot juggle pursuing your interests while also caring for your loved one. It is just not possible.

But on occasion, there are small pockets of time you can work towards your life goals. The caregiving journey is not a steady state.

One of the keys to still growing in your own life's purposes is to remove the box. For example if someone's dream is to open a coffee shop and they can't right now because of their caregiving responsibilities, it is good to ask what is the root of that dream. Is it about welcoming others and practicing hospitality?

The box is the shop but the core desires is serving people in a specific way. This can still be accomplished without the box. Welcoming others and practicing hospitality can be implemented just in other ways.

Or if the desire is to sell coffee as a business, maybe this practice starts to happen from home with packaged coffee instead of in a building. It's the same thing minus the box.

Take another example such as wanting to teach. A person may not have the "box" of a classroom during the season of caregiving but instead can use the core desire of helping others through education. That could then translate into using the windows of time to learn, study and prepare teaching material. Or even to go online to help others in that specific area of interest.

Ask yourself what are your passions and what are their roots. How can you continue to work towards your own life goals and interests just without the traditional box?

Continuing to grow in the direction of your personal purpose matters. You can take the pockets of time to study, learn, prepare, or have a different expression of that purpose.

It may also be a time to delve into some new interests. What are some things you would like to learn and grow in that you haven't had time to do so before? Perhaps taking a class online would be good or just taking some general interest courses that are online and low-commitment.

The reason you want to continue in your area of purpose and interest is to help your emotional energy. It is easier said than done when our loved one's needs are so great, but at the same time we can realize that who you are as a person does not have to be compromised. It just needs to look different for the season you are in.

61

IS DEMENTIA HEREDITARY?

I f you are a descendant of someone who has dementia, the question in the back of many a familial caregiver is, "Will I go through this also?"

There are some notable risk factors such as being over 50 years old, females tend to have it more often, and having a history of dementia or Parkinson's disease in the family may be a contributing factor as well. But there is no guarantee that the next generation will get the disease. There are many things such as a healthy lifestyle that can affect the potential for the disease.

Are there preventative measures?

1) **Hearing Checks** - Oddly enough, those with hearing issues have a significantly higher risk of developing dementia. Most people with hearing problems do not realize they have hearing problems. It is worthy getting your ears checked every 2 years after you turn 45 years of age.

If you need hearing aids, humble yourself. Get them. Use them. They are not cheap. But what is more expensive is early dementia.

2) **Gum Health** - This is another oddity but somehow your gum health is connected to your brain health. Flossing is something we all need to be vigilant about.

3) **General Anesthesia verses a Spinal Block** - Check with your doctor and consult dementia specialists. According to recent studies, if Lewy Body Dementia runs in your family, general anesthesia can be a switch that turns it on but it may be delayed.

Call the Lewy Body Dementia Association for more information and help with talking with your anesthesiologists. By all means get the medical intervention you need. You may just need to do a more careful approach and check out your options.

But there's more than that. Do not let fear be what influences your life.

1) **Live life**. A person never knows when they are going to die and how. Do not wait to fulfill goals and dreams and even as a caregiver, work towards some of those goals.

2) **Do not live in fear**. Fear is very hard on a person's health. Extended fear can actually create problems.

3) **Take care of yourself**. This is easier said than done when you are a caregiver. But always be working towards not just eating healthy and getting proper exercise, but maintaining and growing relationships and dealing with past hurts and harms.

4) **Keep your records updated**. Whether it's from dementia or something else, we will all die. Make sure your financial and legal records as mentioned previously are up-to-date. This can help reduce family stress.

5) **Discuss with your loved ones how you want to be cared for in later life**. Do you prefer to be cared for at home or in a facility? Do you have insurance to assist with this. This is a "just in case" scenario.

At the end of the day, do not let the fear that dementia might come to you stop you in your life aspirations in any way. Nobody can predict what will happen in life. What is most important is to know what you want out of life and always be working towards those goals in small ways and big.

62

PRAY. ASK GOD FOR HELP.

Caregiving has within it a new diagnosis to understand, thousands of decisions to make, working with family and doctors, and trying to figure out what is best for your loved one.

God has a tender place in his heart for the widows, the children and the elderly. He is eager to help those who help those in need, no matter your level of faith.

When you become a caregiver, there are days when you need a miracle just to keep going. Ask for it.

Use this season to nurture your spiritual life.

Read. Discover. Pray.

If it is any comfort Jesus himself experienced caregiving challenges. When Jesus' mother was at the foot of the cross, his brothers and sisters were nowhere around. It is why at the cross he gave his disciple John the responsibility of caring for his mother.

TIPS TO GETTING NECESSARY PAPERWORK COMPLETED

63

FINANCIAL REALITIES

Inflation is exploding around the world and it is getting more and more challenging to cover the costs of living expenses. Not only that but caregiving needs are expensive. There's just no getting around it. But here are some suggestions.

1) <u>Do Anything and Everything to Get Out of Debt</u> - Have garage sales, sell bigger things you don't need, cut monthly subscriptions, etc... Get creative.

2) <u>Use a Budget</u> - Get budgeting software or go it on your own. With money tighter, your awareness of how your money is being spent is critical. It may be a season to "trim the fat."

3) <u>Discover Delivery Driver Services</u> - Going to town? On your way home do a quick delivery. There are a number of delivery services out there - GrubHub, Door Dash, Spark, etc... An extra $50 per week can make a difference just in paying for gas or common items. Or a little more work could equal a car payment.

Do not look at these services less for being a small contribution to your income. If it can help you pay for a tank of gas or a trip to the grocery store, it is worth it.

4) <u>Make your own laundry detergent</u> - Caregiving tends to go through a lot of laundry. In the earlier stages, homemade laundry detergent can work fine. There are resources on the web. Use commercial laundry detergent for the bigger messes that come later on.

5) <u>Do remote work that is not bothered by interruptions</u>. Do know they take a chunk out but the new feature with added tips can help replace some of that.

6) <u>If there are resources in your local government for help, use it if it is appropriate</u>. There can be a lot of stigma for using government resources for help, but at the same time, it is your tax money you paid. It is Ok to get that back in your hour of need.

7) <u>When there is a sale on supplies that you need for caregiving, buy in quantity</u>. This is not always possible, but if you have even just an extra $100, you can save time and money by buying in bulk. This includes not only items such as briefs and other caregiving items, but think of items such as animal food, canned food or other items.

Create a supply closet of extra toiletries, food, and other needs that you know you will need. It's not about becoming a full-on prepper but on getting items you need knowing inflation a year from now will make it more costly.

Life right now is expensive, and it growing more costly every day. Inflation around the world is hurting a lot of people. It isn't going to stop any time soon.

In the past we may have been able to be more relaxed and casual about our financial situations. That time is not now.

Even if you are financially secure, we must all recognize that the world, the banking systems, and the economies are in a very unstable place. Plan accordingly. We have to be smart in how we can take care of our loved ones.

64

LEGAL DOCUMENTS YOU MAY WANT TO COMPLETE

There are legal considerations to consider when a loved one falls ill, and it is better to deal with these prior to the disease progressing. Otherwise, it can create family conflict, could require going before a judge to determine incompetency, and complicate other practical matters.

Many families do not deal with these issues as their loved one does not want to face their own mortality. It can be a sensitivity issue.

Choose someone in the family who has the best relationships with your loved one to ask the difficult questions. Here are forms you may want to think about and questions you probably should ask.

1) <u>Is there a Will in place</u>? - A will is a legal document about how your property, money, and other assets will be distributed upon someone's death. This is usually drawn up by a lawyer. In it make sure it is not just about the passing on of assets, but end-of-life arrangements such as a funeral, how one want to be buried and more. Make sure that the will stays updated and is in a known and accessible place.

2) <u>A Living Trust</u> - This is the naming of the person, a trustee, who will hold and distribute property or manage affairs when the loved one is no longer able to do so.

3) <u>Durable Power of Attorney for Finances</u> - This names someone who can make financial decisions for a loved one when they are no longer able to do so.

You can hire a lawyer to do this or you could print one off on the internet and have it notarized. Check with professionals to see which is best.

4) <u>Durable Power of Attorney for Healthcare</u> - You will need this one as well when they are no longer able to make decisions for themselves. When your loved one has a medical need, your hospital or provider will need a copy of this on record as well as typically a statement from your doctor stating your loved one is no longer able to make medical decisions.

You can hire a lawyer to do this or you could print one off on the internet and have it notarized. Check with professionals to see which is best.

5) <u>Do Not Resuscitate (DNR) Document</u> - This document tells the medical personnel whether your loved one wants to be resuscitated and left on life support, or if in medical need life support measures are to be removed. Your hospital will typically ask if you have these papers.

6) <u>HIPPAA</u> - On hospital records, the person needs to name someone whom a doctor or lawyer can talk to about their needs.

7) <u>Transfer on Death Deed</u> - People tend to think a will is sufficient but after someone passes, if there is only a will for the property deed it will go to probate. This is the legal aspect and requires lawyers and a cost of around $5,000. One way to deal with this is that a lawyer for around $50 can work with your loved one and the benefi-

ciaries to sign a Transfer on Death Deed. This bypasses probate and when someone dies, the deed goes to the persons named. This may require working with the title company but $50 compared to $5000 can be significant.

8) <u>Beneficiaries Named</u> - Do cars and bank accounts have beneficiaries named? These need to be updated.

These are not easy conversations to have with your loved one, but they are important. The better the communication, the greater the peace in the family system.

65

FINANCIAL INFORMATION TO CONSIDER

I f a loved one passes away, are their income, assets, life insurance policies, and other things in place? Where are their bank accounts?

Here are some areas to consider:

- Sources of income (IRA, 401k, investments, bonds, property, etc...)

- Bank accounts - Are the beneficiaries named?

- Social Security Information

- Insurance information (life insurance, long-term care insurance, car and home insurance, etc. Are the agents' names and account numbers listed?

- Is there anything owed anywhere? (Credit cards, liabilities, taxes, etc...) and how much? What are the account numbers?

- The house - Where is the deed, the mortgage held, payments, etc...

- The car - Where are the titles? Are they paid off? Do they have named beneficiaries?

- Are there any safety deposit boxes or keys?

This is a sensitive issue as elder fraud is huge. Loved ones may want to guard this issue because A) They know elder fraud is huge, and B) They may be experiencing the paranoia complex that is associated with dementia in which they accuse loved ones of trying to steal from them.

If there is a potential for fraud, work with an elder attorney. They may be able to work with you to instruct you on how to safeguard your loved one.

66

QUESTIONS TO ASK OTHERS

There are a number of questions to ask the different professionals that can help you with caregiving. Here's a list that is not exhaustive but can stimulate conversation with those to whose help you need.

<u>Elder Lawyers</u>

1) Is the "Will and Testament" of our loved one in place?

2) If our loved one lives for 5+ years or more, what can we do to prepare?

3) If our loved one may pass away sooner, what paperwork do we need in place?

4) Is there a Transfer on Death (TOD) form for the house in place and how does that work if there's a spouse.?

5) Are both medical and financial Power of Attorney forms completed? (These also can be done on your own and notarized).

6) Do we have a DNR (Do Not Resuscitate) form completed if our loved one chooses this option? (You can also do this independently as long as it is desired.)

7) How can we guard against fraud in handling the finances of our loved one?

Physical Therapists

1) Will you teach me the best transfer techniques for the season my loved is currently in?

2) Is there any adaptive equipment that would be best for the season we are in? And will Medicare cover it?

Occupational Therapists

What transfer equipment would you suggest for the season my loved one is currently in?

Doctor

1) Is there medical equipment that we may need that insurance or Medicare will cover?

2) Can we get a prescription for protein drinks?

3) Do you know any resources that can be of assistance to us in our caregiving journey?

Area Council on Aging

1) Is respite care available by the state for caregivers, and if so, how many hours are available?

2) Are there bath aides available and if so, how long can we use that service?

3) Are there food services available to help us out with meals?

4) What other services do you have to help us through this season?

<u>Questions for Your Loved One</u> (To ask with great gentleness and sensitivity on good days only by the best person for the job.)

1) Do you have your will up-to-date? And in place? And where do you keep it?

2) Do you want doctors to attempt resuscitation or not? What about a feeding tube? (Fill out DNR if no).

3) Are you willing to sign a Transfer on Death deed for the transfer of the house?

4) Have you confirmed that your bank accounts have the beneficiaries that you would like?

5) Do the deeds to the car have beneficiaries assigned?

6) Are any life insurance policies up to date?

7) Should you pass away, where do you keep the paperwork for the insurance, deeds and care titles?

8) Whenever you are to pass away, is cremation Ok or do you want to be buried in the traditional way?

9) Where would you like to be buried?

Questions for Family Members

1) How can we all get through this season together so that no one person is heavily burnt out?

2) Are we agreed upon who acts as the trustee of essential decisions?

3) Are we all clear on how our loved one wants to be buried?

4) Are we all clear on the Will per our loved one's wishes?

67
A NURSING FACILITY?

Try as you might, there may come a time when you realize you are no longer able to care for your loved one at home. Sometimes such circumstances arise. Be at peace that you have tried everything in your power for as long as you could.

Search for a good nursing home or small, independent dementia unit. Smaller is definitely better. There are a number of homes that have 10-12 residents that may be more ideal for your loved one's needs.

- Talk to potential homes about their staff/client ratio. If that number is too high, they might not get the level of care that is ideal for your loved one.

- Ask about medical care. Will your loved one be required to take additional medication?

- Ask about social activities. What do they have for those with dementia?

<u>Always</u> take a full tour of the facility. You will learn more from a tour than merely asking questions. Make observations.

- Are their staff kind to the elderly they serve or are they worn out and look haggard?

- Are there sufficient staff available that you observe?

- Does the place have an odor that may be indicative of elders not getting their briefs changed often enough?

- Do they require pandemic vaccination standards? How did they handle the pandemic?

If you decide to go this route, you may notice that the agitation and distress in your loved one increase significantly. They may ask often to go home. It is not an easy transition. Not just for you but for them as well.

When your loved one is placed in a home, it is best to continue to visit them on at least a weekly basis. They still will need your presence. You still matter to them.

Visiting them regularly is not only for their comfort and connection but also so you can see how they are being cared for by the staff. If they are not being appropriately cared for, feel free to talk to those in charge. And if worse comes to worse, you can always take them out and change facilities.

It can be hard for your loved one to change often, so this needs to be taken into consideration. But sometimes you may just need to move your loved one based on the care or lack thereof that they are receiving.

If your loved one is in the final stages and does not respond much, know that what you say and how you say it still matters. As mentioned previously, hearing is one of the last senses to go, even in death. They may not be able to respond, but they can still know and hear your voice. Be loving with your words and discuss sensitive information outside of their hearing, even if it looks like they are unable to hear anything.

On the financial side, paying for a nursing home is expensive. Some people falsely assume they can just have their loved one sign the house over to someone else in the family and then apply for Medicaid. This is generally considered fraud.

Medicaid has a 5-year look-back period to see if there has been any major financial transactions such as the sale of the house, movement of money, etc... This is why it is helpful to consult an elder attorney as to the best course of action.

Sometimes a nursing home becomes a necessity. Life situations can sometimes dictate this. In a perfect world, it is best to keep your loved one home and around family but it isn't always possible. There is space for grace in situations that become too much to bear.

68

TO USE HOSPICE OR NOT

Hospice is a government funded program for those whom a doctor predicts that a patient is in their last 6 months of life. Hospice companies are independent companies that can then serve the family free of charge.

Hospice at the time of this writing traditionally covers

- In home nursing checkups
- Medical supplies and equipment such as lifts and a hospital bed
- Sometimes assistance with cleaning and respite care (adult babysitting)
- Some medications
- Therapy (physical, occupational and speech)n
- Nutrition
- Oxygen services
- Social work services
- Counseling
- Spiritual care

- Grief counseling

It is worth noting that the goal of hospice is not to help your loved one live longer. Their goal is to lead your loved one to the end of life by reducing pain and making their journey more comfortable.

Because of that, there are things that typically are not covered. If your loved one needs IV fluids, a hospital visit and other help that prolong life, it is not likely they will be covered. Or encouraged.

To get those things once has to go off hospice temporarily, then back on, which is not really the goal of hospice. Comfortable end of life is their goal.

Pros and Cons of Hospice

Pros:

- The financial burden of medical supplies is taken care of as hospice tends to cover these expenses

- Pain medication is covered

- There is in-home nursing and care for your loved one so you do not have to leave the house on a regular basis

- There can be a measure of respite care where people will come in and watch your loved one so you can have a rest

- There is help such as grief counseling after your loved one has passed away.

Cons:

- You typically do not retain your current doctor, although they are often informed

- The goal is to walk your loved to the end of life, not help them with certain medical conditions that prolong life. Sometimes this means not getting help you think your loved one might benefit from

- Your way of giving them comfort in their end days may not be their way. It can create a bit of tension.

- Their goal is not prolonged life. And this will show up in how they make recommendations. You ultimately make the decision but you may need to hold your ground on some issues

Your Options:

- You can stop hospice care at any time if it is not a good fit. You are in charge.

- If you do not like the hospice company, you can change to a different company

One of the big things is that in some states, if a person dies and they are not on hospice, it entails a full police investigation upon your loved one's death. This alone can be traumatizing when you are trying to grieve your loss.

How to Aquire a Hospice Company

Look on the internet and talk to your physician about recommended hospice companies. Hospitals typically have particular companies that they work with throughout the duration.

Also look at reviews online. Reviews will matter.

Once you have selected a company, call them and let them know your situation. They will get in touch with your doctor and handle it from there.

Overall the benefits of hospice edge out some of the cons. They can take a burden off of you.

It is an individual decision. The good thing is you are not locked into it. If you find out that it isn't working well for you and your situation, you can stop hospice or change companies.

69
PARTICIPATION IN CLINICAL STUDIES

D ementia is an evolving science. There is so much to learn and new breakthroughs are being made continuously. Yet there is so much more that needs to be discovered.

If your loved one is in early or the mid states of dementia, your loved one may be a good candidate if they are willing to participate in a clinical trial.

What a clinical trial entails is typically exploring how new medicines affect the disease in the brain. There is group that is given the new medicine and another group that is given a placebo. No one knows if they have the real medicine or the placebo.

Regular visits to the researchers occur where doctors examine your loved one. Typically the study is for a certain duration.

At the very least, even if your loved one is not necessarily helped by the trial medication or study, their participation always helps the advancement of research and understanding.

You can check into available clinical trials at https://www.lbda.org/research/clinical-trials/ for Lewy Body Dementia, or Alzheimers.gov for Alzheimer's. Another place you can check is at your local Division 1 medical university if they have a dementia research center.

70

WHAT TO DO WHEN SOMEONE PASSES AWAY

When someone passes away that you care deeply about, you typically want to just be in a quiet space to grieve. But right at the beginning, there are important steps you need to take in handling the affairs of your loved one.

1) Get a legal pronouncement of death.

This is the key to handling all their legal, financial, and practical matters as this will be required to get a death certificate. If your loved one passes away in a nursing home or at a hospital, the staff will usually handle this. Ask how that is taken care of and how you can get it.

If your loved one passes away at home, you still will need a professional to declare their death. This means taking them to the hospital via ambulance where they can be declared deceased. At that point they can then be moved to a funeral home.

If your loved one died while receiving hospice care, a hospice nurse is typically authorized to declare them deceased.

2) <u>Inform relatives, then friends in an appropriate order.</u>

First of all, call those closest in the family to let them know of their death. After that call the friends of the deceased and let them know personally. Honoring the order of closest relationships first is important.

When all immediate family and closest friends have been notified, then group texts or posts on social media can be made to let others know.

You may need to scroll through any lists on their phone or other areas where they may have kept numbers to let others know.

3) <u>Learn about funeral and burial plans and make a choice</u>

This is the time when you talk about the plans, the costs, and more. This may be a family decision especially if there has not been prior discussion.

It is highly advised that matters such as how the person wants to be buried, in the traditional way or through cremation, be discussed prior to reduce familial conflict. Here are some things you will need to consider:

- Which funeral home will you use?

- Do you want cremation or a traditional funeral service?

- If cremation where will the ashes be interred and by whom or if as a group, when?

- If a traditional funeral service, what and who will pick out the tombstone? And where will the burial be located?

- If the person was a veteran will they offer military honors? Call the local VA.

LINDSAY WHITE, CPTA AND DEMENTIA CAREGIVER

The VA may also help not just help with a military salute but can at times help pay for the cost of a headstone and/or engraving.

4) <u>Funeral Service Planning</u>

Decide who will write an obituary, who will be the pallbearers, who will deliver the eulogy, and organize the service. Will there be someone who will collect any gifts received and send out thank you notes at a later date?

If your loved one is being transported to another state the funeral home can help you work this out. If your loved one has been cremated, you will need paperwork to carry with you to cross state lines with the ashes.

If your loved one is buried in a cemetery, you may want to ask what is allowed as far as gifts that can be brought to the tombstone.

5) <u>Property Care</u>

Unfortunately theft after someone dies can happen. Thieves peruse the obituaries. Make sure the house and possessions are secured during funeral times. Have neighbors keep an eye on the house.

Also loved ones may feel the need to go in and take whatever they want, whenever they want, without asking other family members. This can be a point of tension for family. Discuss this together beforehand.

Make sure pets are cared for appropriately.

6) <u>Handling practical matters</u>

Find out what bills need to be paid. What subscriptions need to be cancelled? What credit card or other outstanding debts do they have? Are there recurring bills that need stopped?

7) <u>Get at least 6-8 copies of the Death Certificate</u>

You will need the death certificate to close accounts, file life insurance claims, and handle other matters. You can

work with the funeral home to get these or you can go through your local vital statistics office.

8) Find the Will and work with the Executor

The Executor is the person who manages the settling of the estate in their will. If there isn't a will, a probate court judge will typically name someone.

9) Potentially Hire an Attorney.

You don't have to have one but hiring a lawyer to help navigate the process and distribution of assets may be a more peaceful way to handle family. matters. This is especially true if more than one person is named on the property.

10) Accounting

Depending on the state, a tax return may or may not need to be filed on the estate on behalf of the deceased.

11) Probate Court

Probate is where a will is carried out, but one in which all liabilities are settled first. After that, the remaining assets are then handed over to named beneficiaries.

Some states require a full list of all assets including but not limited to bank accounts, house, cars, personal property, furniture, jewelry, etc... An appraiser can help with this.

12) Contact Social Security if they were Receiving Benefits

The number for the Social Security office is 1-800-772-1213 (www.ssa.gov) or you can contact your local office. The checks will stop coming. Sometimes family may be eligible for some benefits.

Funeral directors can help with contacting Social Security but it is the ultimate responsibility of the remaining family.

13) <u>Contacting Financial Institutions and Closing Accounts</u>

Register with life insurance companies with original death certificates to make a claim.

If your loved one had Long Term Care insurance, they will need to be notified regardless of whether they received benefits from that insurance plan or not.

Banks and other financial institutions will need to be notified.

Let the three major credit bureaus know by sending a death certificate to either Equifax, Experian and TransUnion. This helps prevent identity theft.

Frequent flier points may be transferred to a beneficiary depending on the company if that has been previously set.

14) <u>Cancel their driver's license or ID Card</u>

They too will need a death certificate. They may also need the driver's license or ID. This too helps prevent identity theft.

15) <u>Closing voter registration</u>

County and state voting agencies need notified of death via a death certificate. This helps prevent identity theft for the purposes of voter fraud.

Sound overwhelming? It really can be. There are a lot of details to handle in the midst of great grief.

71

BONUS: MEDICAL EQUIPMENT REVIEW

Q UICK ACCESS: For a sharable document that has all the links for easy clicking, please go to https://bit.ly/dememtiaequipmentlinks

Medical equipment is almost always necessary and what you need will change throughout the journey. Here are some honest thoughts on various equipment.*

General Accessories

DIY ID & Medical Alert Card - https://amzn.to/3rucqH2 - This is an important card for your loved one's purse or wallet.

Food/Freezer Plates for Make Ahead Cooking - https://amzn.to/44abBB6 - Caregiving can be exhausting but if you take one day a week and cook extra meals, they can be placed in the freezer and microwaved for later. This can be helpful not just for you but respite care workers or other carers who come in to assist.

DeChoker - https://amzn.to/3phw2NM - Choking can be life-threatening for those with dementia. This can be a helpful tool to keep on hand.

Neck Pillow - https://amzn.to/3J3vYI8 - This is a very helpful product to reduce the Lewy lean and lessen neck strain. It does not fully take care of the issue but it is a help.

Pager Call Button - https://amzn.to/3MZpif1 - This can help your loved one, especially at night to call you if needed.

Motion Sensor and Pager - https://amzn.to/3MUMlb3 - Roaming can be an issue. And at night this especially be a problem. A motion sensor will help alert you when there is a need for intervention. Another option that gives alerts on your phone: https://amzn.to/3XjIadA

Spice Rack for a Pill Organizer - https://amzn.to/465QiCC - Sometimes love ones have a lot of pills to take and the traditional snap-top pill holders do not work. Spice racks on the other hand work. Put pills in the bottles and they can easily become grab-and-go. Here are some bottles that can be used https://amzn.to/42zZagC

Transfer Equipment

Black gait belt - https://amzn.to/43Hc11O - This doesn't scream "gait belt" so much but can blend in typically with what they are wearing.

Collapsible Single Point Cane - https://amzn.to/3P3Wchw - This can be used at very early stages. Although it may just be best to start with a quad cane.

Quad Cane - https://amzn.to/3CkgJa0 - A great tool in the early stages. Easy to use and can be adjusted to both left or right hands. What is most handy is it stands up on its own.

Four Wheel Walker - https://amzn.to/3qsZRuN - These are very standard to use in the early stages and can be a place for your loved one to sit and rest.

Front Wheel Walker - https://amzn.to/43Q4bD2 - When balance begins to change, this is the next in the mobility progression.

No Wheel Walker - https://amzn.to/3qt0swx - This is more stable but it can also be more difficult for a loved one to maneuver.

Tennis Balls for Walker - https://amzn.to/43udmJv - You can make your own but you can buy these already done for you.

Lightweight collapsible wheelchair - https://amzn.to/45QackJ - This chair is great on concrete but not so great over any other variable terrain.

Bed railing - https://amzn.to/3qqBCxk - This can be used to prevent rolling out of bed prior to getting a hospital bed. It just slides under the mattress.

Foam Elevation Pad for Bed - https://amzn.to/3WZcM47 - An elevated foam pad can be used for better breathing and sleeping. This can be true if they have sleep apnea issues or choking. Consult a doctor to see if this is a good fit.

Spin disk for transfers - https://amzn.to/43MDPSj - When your loved one's legs do not take steps as easily, this can be used for basic transfers. Get training in how to safely use these. This one is way more expensive but can also be more effective: https://amzn.to/3NhAuFo. Use a gait belt always.

Get-U-Up Lift - https://amzn.to/3oUluUw - If your loved one cannot use their legs anymore to assist with transfers, this lift can make the difference between keeping your loved home or not. It's easy to use even in late stages.

Toileting and Shower Aids

Toilet Rail System - https://amzn.to/3CgMFMi - This is a simple railing system that can be installed to help give your loved one added hand holds.

Elevated Toilet Seat - https://amzn.to/45VVMiY - These are especially helpful if your loved one has a hip fracture.   It can stain a bit so be sure to keep it clean at all times.

Drop Arm Commode - https://amzn.to/3P2QZpX - This is a great tool for a bedside commode and generally speaking, can be used as a shower bench depending on the size of your loved one.

Bed pan - https://amzn.to/3X3RSkk - Bed pans after a surgery may be needed. Sometimes smaller ones can be Ok and sometimes not. Again, this depends on the size of your loved one.

Shower bench - https://amzn.to/3WZl77y - This is an ideal shower bench that goes both inside and outside of the shower and has adjustable legs.

Swivel Scooting Shower Bench - https://amzn.to/43vpHwT - This shower bench helps with swivel and scooting

Shower railing bar - https://amzn.to/42utucr - These can be used with showering. It is best if they are secured to a wall with nails.

Car Assists

Car Handle Assist - https://amzn.to/45WrCMA - These are great to assist with car transfers and can easily be placed and taken out.

Steering Wheel Car Tray - https://amzn.to/3P2FH51 - In later stages entering and exiting a restaurant may be too much. This tray can help facilitate still eating out but with a "table" in your car to help. This tray is something you can use for much more even beyond elder care if you work out of your car. It is a great asset.

Miscellaneous:

Elder Tracker - Watch kind - https://amzn.to/3CkHUl6 - Waterproof kind - https://amzn.to/3Nu9UsV - If your loved one wanders, an elder tracker is something to seriously consider.

Tell Me Your Story Journal - https://amzn.to/3JfLHnp - This is a guided journal to help record the stories of your loved ones when they are in a good place to talk.

———

The author of this book cannot vouch for the safety, durability or whether this equipment is a good match for your loved one. The quality of the product is a decision between you as the purchaser and the manufacturer, not the author. Ask professionals as to which pieces of equipment, how to use it, how to fit it for your loved and what is best used for your situation. The same is true for all service recommendations as well.

72

BONUS: WEBSITES AND RESOURCES

Y‌ou are not alone. There are resources available that can help you along the way. You will do well to learn what these resources offer and how they can be of assistance.

Lewy Body DementiaAssociation (lbda.org)- This is one of the main websites dedicated specifically to this form of dementia. They also can be a good resource to call when needing to navigate special situations such as during hospital stays. If you sign up for the mailing list, they can also let you know when there are clinical trials in which you might be able to participate in to help advance research.

Eldercare Locator

800-677-1116

https://eldercare.acl.gov

The eldercare locator is a website where you type in your zip code and it will give you several community resources specific to your area. This is a very valuable tool and worth the time to look into.

Alzheimer's Disease.gov

www.Alzheimers.gov

This website has some very helpful resources. They also occasionally announce clinical trials in which you and your loved one can participate in.

Caregiver

www.caregiver.com

This website has some conferences, magazines and other helpful articles.

Robin's Wish - A movie? Yes. Sometimes we can find encouragement in the journey of others. This is the story of Robin William's bout with dementia, although his family and friends really didn't know his diagnosis at the time. https://amzn.to/3pOl8vN

73
BONUS: SUPPORT GROUPS

The caregiving journey is just a challenging journey. Relationships are messy. Taking care of your loved one is messy. And navigating all the ins and outs of dementia is messy.

1) <u>During the Caregiving Journey</u>

One resource you may want to access is support groups specific to dementia. There are also support groups for dementia in general.

Some of these support groups are not just in person but can also be online. Check out the Alzheimer's Association for trained professional groups at https://www.alz.org/

2) <u>After your loved one has passed away</u>

Grief happens not just because a loved one has passed away, but often it is about the whole package of grieving changed relationships, familial pressures, financial challenges, and the whole journey.

There are support groups focused on navigating grief. Many churches and social organizations offer such groups. You can find grief groups in your area by putting your zip code into this web search:

www.griefshare.com

Grief is a journey that is very unique to every person. We never know how we are going to grieve.

There are also professional counselors that can help you to navigate the grieving process. Grief is real and having someone help you through the process can make a difference in your healing journey.

Why get help with grief? By taking the time to grieve well, it empowers your heart to once again love well.

74
CRUCIFIED LOVE OF THE CAREGIVER

Those black circles under my eyes?
They're not pretty to you,
but they're actually halos of love.
Not the mushy, starry-eyed kind
but the love that says I'll do what it takes
to love her with all I have.

That fragrance you smell when I'm around?
It's not pleasant to you,
but it's actually a very expensive perfume.
It may smell like urine and not having showered enough,
but it's the smell of love that says I'll do anything
to love her even if I get soiled.

That messy house that you no longer visit?
It's not proper to you,
but it's actually a glorious cathedral.
Not the kind that has stained glass windows
and vaulted ceilings,

but the cathedral of love that says I'll give my best
to love her most.

Those words that you hear?
They're not patient enough for you,
but they're actually beautiful music.
Not the kind with violins and drums
but the kind that says I'll do what it takes
to protect her heart and life from harm.

This love that I talk about?
It's not always doable, even for me,
but my effort to live it is heaven's joy.

And it IS the kind that comes with angel's songs
and tambourines
to the glory of one who is love to me.

75
MY MOTHER IN THE MEN'S ROOM

I took my mother far into the men's room today,
not because I'm making a political statement but
because as her caregiving daughter,
I'm sleep-deprived.

I walked out of the store the other day without paying,
not because I wanted to take something
(I immediately went back in)
but because as her caregiving daughter,
I was livid with anger at someone who is opposing us.

I snapped at my mother the other day
when she tried to sit on a chair of air,
not because I wanted to be mean to her but
because as her caregiving daughter,
I wanted her to be safe, again.

"Take time for yourself," they said.

I went to a movie and all I could think of was
wanting to be with her.
During the 12 times a night she calls me
I can't say no to her heart-breaking cries.

"Take care of yourself," they said.
"Take care of yourself."
It's a good word of wisdom. But...

Do they realize the only free time
I have I want to sleep?
Do they realize
I don't have the emotional energy to
"put myself out there?"
Do they realize what it takes to do this?

They don't. And it's Ok.

Because I don't realize the level of their hurts,
pains, and hardships either.
My past insensitive words to them
have more than likely been on the same level
as their words to me.

Grace.

To them. To me. To the world.

It's better than time.

Time would be nice, but I don't always have it.

But grace? That's a choice.

A choice I can give to myself that
lightens the burden of obligations.
A gift I can give to others when they say and
do what is not needed.
A well of life when I confront decisions that
I don't want to make but feel are necessary.

When I was about five
I stopped my mother from going into the men's room.
Now that I'm an adult she returned the favor.

After we got out of there, quick, we laughed.

We were graced.

ABOUT THE AUTHOR

Lindsay White has been a full-time dementia caregiver with more than 10 years of experience. This unexpected journey began first for her grandmother with Alzheimer's, and in the last decade with her mother who had Lewy Body Dementia.

Lindsay knows well the path of getting a diagnosis to an unknown and mysterious disease with many unusual behaviors. Her goal is to help others along this journey by equipping them with fundamental skills and knowledge in an easy-to-access format.

ABOUT THE AUTHOR

WILL YOU HELP?

Will You Help Others?

If you have learned something helpful, please leave your feedback on Amazon. Why?

1) Amazon mainly promotes books with reviews. Without them, helpful books like this will get lost in the Amazon jungle.

2) It is incredibly encouraging! And if you are a caregiver, you know that encouragement is like a drop of water in a parched land.

Thank you,

Lindsay White

www.ingramcontent.com/pod-product-compliance
Lightning Source LLC
LaVergne TN
LVHW051551080426
835510LV00020B/2949